UNLOCKING

THE CODE OF

UNLIMITED

POTENTIAL

24 Spiritual Insights and Transformational Practices

To Unlock a Life of Miracles and Awaken The Limitless Potential Within

Ioana Aura Munteanu

Note to the reader: This book is intended as an informational guide. The approaches, perspectives and techniques described herein are meant to supplement, and not to be a substitute for professional medical care or treatment. They should not be used to treat a serious ailment without prior consultation with a qualified health care professional.

Quantum science suggests
that every moment
holds within it countless possible futures,
each waiting to be awakened by the choices we make
today.

Ancient wisdom echoes
a profound truth:
we are here for one purpose above all—to love.

This book is dedicated
to guiding you on a journey of rediscovering this
love,
tapping into your inherent power to create
heaven on earth.

TABLE OF CONTENTS

FOREWORD

Each of us has the potential to experience boundless love, profound peace, true freedom, vibrant health—all the ultimate desires of the human spirit. When we fully grasp and remember our limitless inner power, when we rediscover the extraordinary strength and beauty within ourselves, these aspirations become more than dreams—they become our reality.

We can all sense the accelerating pace of the world around us, the profound changes, and the rapid shifts unfolding in every aspect of our lives. As a result, many have been called to share their spiritual awareness and become beacons of light, guiding other to make the profound shift from fear to love.

Their radiant presence has helped many of us come closer to the light that has always patiently resided within us. There is a powerful call for lightworkers, and we have the potential to be part of this new wave. We have the ability to be a lighthouse—not only for ourselves but also for others.

The key to this transformation lies in a simple but profound shift: moving from the illusion of fear to the truth of love. While this may seem like a monumental step, it becomes

1

less daunting when taken moment by moment, especially as we navigate the complexities of daily life in this world. However, it is essential that we take full responsibility for the life we are living right now. By doing so, we empower ourselves to gather the tools, wisdom, and strength needed to awaken spiritually and manifest the life we truly desire.

We have the power to shift deep-rooted patterns in areas such as relationships, health, work, finances, and spirituality, replacing them with a renewed commitment to awareness. By examining every aspect of our lives that feels in need of change, we can begin the process of clearing our blocks—starting with the crucial step of recognizing them.

Clarity is a powerful force, and once we gain it, it will guide us to the right tools and practices needed for our unique lessons at the perfect time. Listen to your soul, trust your inner wisdom, and apply the tools that resonate with you. Above all, never forget that we are always being guided, always being watched over, and always being supported on this journey.

The 24 spiritual insights and transformational practices found in this book offer powerful tools to embrace your journey, cultivate presence, expand your awareness, and tap into profound joy. In a world craving accessible wisdom, these bite-sized portions of timeless truth are designed to be revisited time and again, providing guidance to connect with our purest spiritual essence.

In various spiritual traditions, the number 24 symbolizes divine protection and guidance, harmony between material and spiritual realms, and the completion of transformative cycles. Each of these 24 themes carries the potential to reinforce your spiritual identity and draw you closer to a miraculous life of love, joy, and freedom. These universal desires are within each of us—sometimes dormant yet waiting patiently for us to rediscover or remember them. Through these practices, we can reclaim our highest potential, and then, moving further on our spiritual evolution, we can shift from *"doing"* to just *" being"*.

Using this book, you will learn to recognize the vast, untapped potential within yourself, reimagine the boundaries of what is possible and learn that the idea of *"unlimited"* is not a far-off ideal but a natural extension of who you are. Through its pages, you are encouraged to explore the infinite dimensions of your being, breaking free from the constraints of old perceptions and reconnecting with the boundless nature of your true self.

Each chapter in this book weaves together spiritual principles, tools, and practices that illuminate this truth: that miracles, magic, and boundless potential are natural to us when we reconnect with our inner strength and awaken our true nature. By engaging with the spiritual principles, tools and practices within these pages, you will reconnect with the richness of your spiritual identity and ignite daily miracles. This journey invites you to see yourself not merely as part of the natural world, but as a creator capable of profound transformation and a deeply fulfilling life.

In nearly 25 years of spiritual exploration, guided by lessons from Yoga, Reiki, the Akashic Records, channeling, meditation practices and dedicated study of the wisdom of spiritual masters, I have uncovered profound spiritual experiences that have reawakened my own true power.

As a glimpse into my spiritual journey, I can share that my life was foretold and saved by a priest who appeared to my mother in a powerful dream, changing my destiny even before I was born. As testimony to an unseen protection, by the age of seven I had already survived three near-death experiences—I choked on a candy, was electrocuted, and nearly drowned in the strong current of a river—but I was spared any serious consequences.

These early experiences, along with many others that followed, triggered powerful spiritual awakenings and led me down transformative paths, opening the way to a deeper self-understanding and personal transformation. I began to understand that the boundaries between the physical and the spiritual are much thinner than most people realize, and that we each hold the key to unlocking the supernatural potential that resides within us all. They also taught me to *remember*— to remember that we are all connected to something far greater than ourselves, something that exists beyond the physical realm.

To be able to manifest what we want in life, we have to be open to receive and willing to receive when the opportunity or life's lessons appears. Often, over the years of our lives, we have installed defences, barriers, or walls inside ourselves. These walls are mechanism to feel safe, but many times they shut out desired influences, such as growth, friendship, intimacy, or love. An essential step in making our desires possible is to soften these barriers enough to let those lessons go inside us when they show up.

Another obstacle to our receptivity is to believe that we must be aggressive in order to get what we want. This type of belief will trigger a tunnel vision, and we will fail to see the opportunities. Softening our defences and becoming willing to remain open to possibilities outside our immediate real of vision can shift in an opposite direction our luck and destiny.

If we are looking for new opportunities, new friendships, new love, new expansion, we might first look within ourselves to see where we are shut down. We need to become more open as individual and more vision expansive. We have to be ready to receive all tools available and all help guided by the universe towards us. We need to believe and have faith that miraculous events are possible, and then be alert and, most importantly, be open to receive and step into extraordinary.

I invite you to step forward with an open heart and mind, embracing the wisdom that resonates with your soul, your true *Essence.* This wisdom has whispered to my heart across many lifetimes and has guided me deeply throughout this journey in this lifetime.

Working on ourselves is one step on the journey, a phase of growth and transformation. But as we ascend to higher levels of awareness, we move beyond the notion of *"work."* At this point, life becomes a dance—fluid, effortless, and in perfect harmony with the flow of the universe. Yet, as we rise even further, we realize that there is no longer any dance, no separation, no need for effort. In this state, there is no time or space to measure; there is only the profound experience of *what is.* It is an eternal, boundless presence—pure, unblemished *Love.*

This *Love* is all-encompassing, beyond form and concept, and it is the very essence of our being. At the highest level, everything simply is, and in that profound stillness, we return to the truth of who we have always been – *Pure Love.*

"To be fully alive, fully human, and completely awake is to be continually thrown out of the nest. "[1]

—*Pema Chödrön*

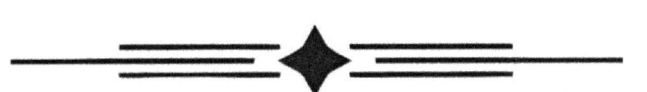

CHAPTER 1

THE UNIVERSAL MIRROR: HEALING WITHIN, HEALING WITHOUT

The world today feels chaotic, as though every institution and belief system are unraveling before our eyes. From the cracks appearing in the structures of religion, economy, and healthcare, to the individual crises of identity many of us are experiencing, it seems as if we're collectively spiraling into darkness.

Beneath this apparent chaos lies a profound spiritual transformation. What we are witnessing is not a collapse for its own sake, but the dissolution of the false self—both on a personal and societal level.

The false self is the construct we build to protect ourselves from the traumas of our past. It begins in childhood when, in moments of pain or rejection, we unconsciously create a persona to shield us from further harm. A child who was punished for failure might become an overachiever, driven by the fear of disappointing others. Another who felt neglected might develop a pattern of codependency, constantly seeking external validation. These coping mechanisms shape our sense of identity, but they are built on fear, not truth.

The Masks We Wear

As adults, we carry these patterns forward, mistaking them for who we are. We become the achiever, the avoider, the pleaser, or the rebel—labels that we identify with so deeply that they obscure our true essence. Over time, this false self extends beyond individuals, embedding itself into societal systems and institutions, which reflect the same patterns of control, fear, and scarcity.

But now, a shift is occurring. The light of consciousness is expanding, forcing us to confront these illusions. Just as sunlight streaming through a window illuminates' dust in the air, the rising awareness in the world is exposing the shadows within us. Trauma, limiting beliefs, and conditioned patterns are coming to the surface, not to punish us, but to be seen, acknowledged, and healed. This illumination is the universal mirror—reflecting our inner struggles and inviting us to heal within, so that healing can manifest outwardly.

For many, this process feels like a death. If we believe we are the false self, its collapse can be terrifying. We may experience depression, anxiety, or even existential dread as the structures we relied on—both internally and externally—begin to crumble.

But this is not an end; it is a beginning. What feels like destruction is, in fact, a birth. Just as we experience inner collapse, we are shown the way out—through introspection, self-awareness, and release, helping us to heal and transform the inner chaos into clarity.

The false self must dissolve to make way for the true self—the divine essence within each of us that is free, expansive, and deeply connected to the present moment.

Unlike the false self, which operates out of fear and scarcity, the true self thrives in love, creativity, and abundance. It does not react to life but flows with it, guided by intuition and an unshakable sense of purpose. This is the light that exists within all of us, the true self that is waiting to be uncovered as we heal the distortions within.

The Collapse of Societal Structures

"It is no measure of health to be well-adjusted to a profoundly sick society."[2] – Krishnamurti

This transformation is not limited to individuals. Institutions built on the energy of the false self—control, manipulation, and profit at the expense of humanity and the planet—are also being exposed. Their cracks are not signs of failure but of a necessary breakdown, paving the way for systems rooted in authenticity, collaboration, and sustainability. This collapse mirrors the individual journey: as we heal and shed our false selves, we collectively create space for a more authentic, compassionate world.

To navigate this shift, we must embrace the discomfort of letting go. This means allowing old patterns to surface, not resisting them, and recognizing that they are not who we truly are. It means questioning the motives behind our actions: *Are we building our lives on fear, or are we guided by love? Are we reacting to old wounds, or are we creating from a place of wholeness?* In this process, the universal mirror serves to reflect the truths we may have been avoiding, helping us to let go of the masks that have obscured our authentic self.

The Alchemy of Transformation: Turning Fear into Light

The path to the true self requires courage, patience, and a willingness to sit with the discomfort of transformation. It is a process of alchemy, where the dense energies of fear and trauma are transmuted into the light of awareness and love.

As we release the false self, we create space for our true essence to emerge, a self that is radiant and limitless. This transformation, both individual and collective, represents the healing of our inner and outer worlds, as we align with the light that mirrors our highest truth.

In a world that seems to be falling apart, this perspective offers hope. The cracks we see, both within ourselves and in society, are not signs of failure but of evolution. The light is expanding, and though it may feel uncomfortable to confront the shadows it reveals, this process is necessary for our collective awakening.

When we start to let go of who we thought we were, we make room for who we truly are. And as more of us step into this authentic self, we will co-create a world that reflects the light within us—a world of compassion, connection, and boundless possibility. The universal mirror reflects the truth of who we are—both individually and collectively. By healing within, we align with our highest potential and create the world we are meant to live in.

This structure creates a natural flow between the concepts, showing how personal transformation and societal shifts are deeply interconnected. The universal mirror offers a guiding principle for both inner healing and collective evolution, helping us recognize that healing within ourselves contributes to the healing of the world around us.

Practice: Releasing the False Self and Embracing the True Self

In a world marked by upheaval and transformation, the concept of the universal mirror reminds us that our inner and outer worlds are deeply interconnected. The chaos we see in society reflects the unresolved patterns within us, and by healing ourselves, we contribute to the collective evolution of humanity.

These practices are designed to help you dissolve the false self, embrace your true essence, and align with the light of authenticity.

As you engage with these practices, you'll discover how personal transformation radiates outward, creating ripples of healing and change in the world around you.

Practices for Letting Go of Illusions and Discovering Your Authentic Self

Self-Inquiry Journaling

Explore your inner patterns by asking reflective questions:

What fears or limiting beliefs are driving my decisions?

Where in my life am I wearing a mask to gain approval or avoid rejection?

What would my life look like if I acted from a place of authenticity?

Body Awareness Practice

Notice where you feel tension or discomfort in your body during moments of stress. Place your hands on these areas and breathe deeply, imagining the tension dissolving into light. This helps release stored trauma and reconnects you with your true self.

Letting Go Ritual

Write down a behavior, belief, or label that no longer serves you on a piece of paper. Reflect on how it has shaped your identity, then burn the paper (safely) or tear it up as an act of release, symbolizing the dissolution of the false self.

Practices for Reflecting Inner Transformation in the Outer World

Mirror Meditation

Sit in front of a mirror and gaze into your eyes. Acknowledge the emotions that arise and affirm: *I see you. I honor your journey. I love the truth of who you are.* This helps you connect with your authentic self beyond the masks.

Conscious Questioning

In moments of doubt or reactivity, pause and ask:

Am I reacting from an old wound, or am I responding from a place of love?

What does my highest self want to create in this situation?

Nature Reflection

Spend time observing nature—trees shedding their leaves, the flow of a river, or the resilience of the seasons. Reflect on how nature mirrors the process of release and renewal, offering guidance for your own transformation.

Practices for Collective Healing Through Inner Transformation

Compassionate Awareness Exercise

When you notice societal issues that feel overwhelming or unjust, instead of reacting with frustration, sit quietly and ask:

How do these issues reflect patterns within me?

How can I cultivate change in my own life that contributes to healing this issue?

This practice turns frustration into purposeful action.

Daily Acts of Authenticity

Commit to one action each day that reflects your true self. It could be speaking your truth in a conversation, creating something meaningful, or simply allowing yourself to rest. Over time, these actions reinforce authenticity and inspire others to do the same.

These practices invite you to embrace transformation, release old patterns, and align with your highest self.

As you step into your truth, you'll notice the ripples of this shift extending outward, fostering authenticity, compassion, and light in your relationships, communities, and beyond. Together, through our individual journeys of healing, we co-create a world that reflects our collective potential—a world grounded in love, connection, and possibility.

"God is the hidden self in every person. "[3]

—Paramahansa Yogananda

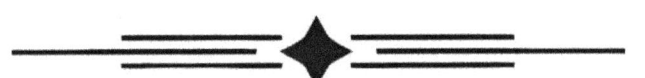

CHAPTER 2

BEYOND THE VEIL: A SOUL'S JOURNEY OF REMEMBRANCE AND RECONNECTION

The *veil* it is known as a metaphorical barrier that separates the physical world from the spiritual realm. It challenges conventional wisdom and questions the limitations of human perceptions, inviting us to look beyond and explore the deeper truths that lie within. The veil is a testimony that our souls are immortal and that in the spiritual realms there is no time, and past, present, and future exist simultaneously.

There are two distinct mindsets that shape our experiences in life: the growth mindset and the reset mindset.

The growth mindset focuses on the belief that our abilities can be developed through dedication, learning from mistakes, and perceiving challenges as opportunities for personal growth. It encourages continuous effort, patience, and long-term development.

However, the reset mindset takes this further. It is the willingness to completely reinvent oneself, to adapt quickly to changing circumstances, to reframe feedback, and to focus on transformational change. It's a dynamic process of reprogramming your inner being—biohacking your consciousness—so that you can awaken your true potential.

It is widely known that most people only use a small fraction of their mental capacity. Some theories suggest that a mere 1% of the population taps into extraordinary abilities or ascends to their highest state of being. Yet, the idea of human potential is constantly being redefined. We are capable of far more than we realize, but this requires conscious leadership of our lives, authenticity, and above all, love. The love we cultivate for others and, most importantly, for ourselves.

The Soul's Journey of Reconnection

Before we are born, our soul has the opportunity to review its future life in collaboration with spiritual guides. In this pre-birth experience, the soul chooses its parents, community, life circumstances, and even the challenges that will shape its earthly journey.

The veil is the term used to describe the limitations we experience when we descend into physical form on Earth. It represents the forgetting of our higher knowing and connection with *Source* that we carried before birth. In the human experience, the veil feels like a dense and restrictive force. Our souls, vast and infinite, must adjust to the constraints of the physical body, which can feel limiting and cold. This veil of forgetfulness causes a disconnect from the boundless wisdom and joy of our higher selves.

However, this life is not about failure—it is about learning and growing through every challenge and every moment. By understanding this truth, we begin to transcend this concept, moving from separation to *Oneness*. Life on Earth is not a linear journey of success and failure; rather, it is a process of evolution.

The veil may obscure our true nature, but it cannot erase it. Every experience—every challenge, triumph, and setback—is part of the divine plan for the soul's evolution. As we grow and awaken, we reconnect with our true nature, remembering that we are not just human beings, but divine souls on a sacred journey. When we embrace the human experience, including the *veil* that comes with it, we learn to transcend fear and reconnect with the divine essence within us.

The human experience is temporary, a passing phase of separation. But the truth is that we are always connected to the *Source* and this forgetfulness may obscure this truth, but it is never lost. As we remember and awaken, we realize that we are always whole, always complete, always loved.

This process of awakening is not just personal but collective. More and more people are beginning to awaken to their true essence, rising in consciousness, and connecting with their higher selves. This shift in consciousness is part of a collective return to *Oneness*. As this illusion begins to lift, we realize that we are all interconnected, all part of the same divine energy.

Throughout history, countless spiritual teachers have spoken of the path of awakening, the journey of transcending the *veil*, and the remembrance of our true essence. Whether it is *Buddha*'s teachings of mindfulness and enlightenment, *Jesus'* messages of love and forgiveness, or the wisdom of *Native American elders*, each of them have pointed to the same truth: we are all divine beings having a human experience, and the ultimate goal is to return to oneness with the *Source*.

Moving Toward Oneness

"We are not human beings having a spiritual experience. We are spiritual beings having a human experience."[4]*— Teilhard de Chardin*

As we grow in awareness and begin to reconnect with our higher selves, we find that the veil is no longer a barrier. It becomes an opportunity for deep, transformative growth. Through this process, we experience life in a more profound way, understanding that we are always connected to the *Source*, that we were never separate, and that the separation we experienced was simply part of the human journey.

The truth of our essence is vast, boundless, and infinite. The more we awaken to this truth, the more we step into our true potential, and the more we see that the *veil* was never real. It was simply a temporary experience designed to help us remember who we truly are.

Practice: Moving Beyond the Veil of Illusion

Stepping beyond the veil is a journey of rediscovering your true nature, reconnecting with your higher self, and remembering that you are a divine being having a human experience. It only represents the illusion of separation—a temporary forgetting of your soul's vastness and oneness with the universe.

This sacred forgetting allows you to grow, learn, and evolve through the challenges and joys of human life. It invites you to awaken, transcend, and step into the fullness of who you are— a multi-dimensional being of love, peace, and power.

The practices below are designed to help you remember your divine essence and reconnect with the limitless potential within you.

Daily Soul Connection

Spend time each day in meditation or prayer. Sit quietly, close your eyes, and focus on your breath. Visualize a golden light connecting you to the universe and your higher self. Feel the love and wisdom of your soul flowing into your heart. Affirm: *I am connected to the infinite love and wisdom of the Source.*

Embrace Challenges as Lessons

When faced with difficulties, remind yourself that they are part of your soul's growth. Journal about the lessons hidden in your experiences and reflect on how these challenges are shaping you into a stronger, wiser version of yourself

Practice Self-Love

Stand in front of a mirror each day and speak kind words to yourself. Affirm: *I am worthy of love, joy, and abundance.* Celebrate your progress, forgive your mistakes, and nurture your body, mind, and soul.

Release Attachments

Reflect on relationships, beliefs, and habits that no longer serve your higher purpose. Set the intention to let them go with love and gratitude. Trust that by creating space, you allow the universe to bring in what aligns with your soul's journey.

Align With Your Soul's Purpose

Spend time identifying your core values and passions. Ask yourself: *What lights me up? How can I serve others while staying true to myself?*

Take small, aligned actions every day to live in harmony with your soul's mission.

Bio-hack Your Consciousness

Explore techniques like mindfulness, gratitude practices, and affirmations to elevate your state of being. Engage in activities like yoga, breathwork, or sound healing to integrate mind, body, and spirit. Nourish your brain and body with healthy foods and restorative sleep.

Cultivate Presence

Practice being fully in the moment. Whether you're washing dishes, walking in nature, or talking to a loved one, bring your attention fully to the experience. Let go of the past and future; the present moment is where life unfolds.

Affirmation:

I am a radiant soul on a journey of remembrance. I am always connected to the Source of love and wisdom. I release fear and embrace my divine potential. I am one with the universe.

With each step you take, remember that every moment is an invitation to reconnect with your true self. The veil is lifting, and you are awakening. Step boldly into your potential, for the journey beyond this illusion is a journey home.

As you practice reconnecting with your essence, you'll begin to realize that the veil was never permanent—it was simply a tool for growth. The challenges and separations you experienced were opportunities to remember your strength, rediscover your purpose, and reconnect with the *Universal Source.*

You were meant to shine. By stepping beyond this boundary, you are not only rediscovering your own light but also inspiring others to do the same.

The journey is not just personal—it is collective, a shared remembrance of the *Oneness* we all came from and to which we will return.

"It is not the strongest of the species that survives, nor the most intelligent; it is the one most adaptable to change"[5]

—Charles Darwin

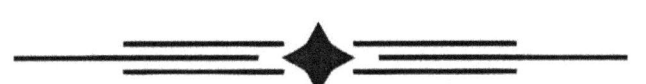

CHAPTER 3

CHANGE IS A CONSTANT: EMBRACING GROWTH AND RESILIENCE

Change is a constant in life. As *Charles Darwin* once said, survival is not determined by the strongest or the most intelligent species, but by those who are most responsive to change. Whether change comes quickly or gradually, it always seeks to strike a balance between the old and the new. Even when change appears slow at first, the eventual outcome can be unimaginable.

Someone starting a meditation practice may feel like nothing is changing at first. They sit in silence, feeling distracted, restless, and unsure if it's making any difference. Over time, as they continue with the practice, they notice moments of calmness, clarity, and a deeper connection with themselves. Eventually, meditation becomes a tool for inner peace, helping them navigate life with more grace and mindfulness than they ever anticipated.

Change is often accompanied by fear. Fear exists on the opposite side of love, and along with worry, can have a deeply harmful impact on our spiritual, personal, and professional growth. The most powerful step we can take is to avoid dwelling on negative thoughts, confront our fears directly, and take calculated risks. By managing fear, we often find ourselves surprisingly bold, able to move forward faster, and with greater clarity, toward our goals.

The Shift in Collective Consciousness

Many of us are increasingly waking up to the realization that the lives we've built no longer align with our expectations or desires. This shift may be due to changes occurring within us over time or as part of the larger transformation affecting all of humanity. Change is unfolding so rapidly that predicting what the future holds has become nearly impossible. As a result, many of the old ways of planning and structuring our lives no longer seem relevant.

If we continue to hold onto outdated patterns, we may find ourselves feeling out of sync with the reality around us. By tuning into the energies shifting in the world, we begin to question beliefs and ideas that, just a few years ago, seemed perfectly logical. At its core, the shift we are experiencing now is about recognizing that we are more than just human. We are multidimensional beings, and our physical, earthly selves are only a small fraction of who we truly are.

As we awaken to this truth, the life we once envisioned for a limited version of ourselves no longer aligns with our reality. For some, this realization unfolds gradually, while for others, it hits like a bolt of lightning. Each of us must find our own path and pace, discovering the way that allows us to integrate this expanded sense of self into our life journey.

Sometimes a drastic change feels totally right, and overnight we might decide to make changes in our life. Other times, we allow the changes to proceed slowly. We may begin with allowing ourselves to dream of a new life or ask the deeper questions that encourage us to discover our true purpose in life. Whatever is the way or the speed of this integration, this entire process is a natural sign of the growth we are all going through. Trust it to guide you to the life of your dreams.

The Transformative Power of Words

Our words—both towards ourselves and others—hold significant power, and reshaping our approach to communication in relationships is key to unlocking its full potential. To truly harness the power of effective and positive communication, we must take action, persevere through challenges, and overcome obstacles. Staying motivated and committed to our personal goals requires consistent effort. In time, this effort becomes rewarding and even addictive as we begin to feel our entire being—body, mind, and soul—transforming and growing stronger with each step.

Our thoughts, when directed with intention, can influence the experiences we attract. Maintaining harmony in our thoughts helps bring harmony into our lives. Using our imagination to visualize success and innovative solutions encourages thinking beyond conventional boundaries, opening doors to new possibilities.

Embracing Chaos as a Catalyst for Growth

"All great changes are preceded by chaos. "[6] *- Deepak Chopra*
In these moments, staying calm amid challenges is crucial. I've found that my most significant transformations and deepest life lessons often arose from those so-called *"dark nights of the soul."* These are the moments when we initially feel defeated and helpless. However, the quicker we take ownership of our role in the situations we face, the sooner we can ground ourselves and shift our focus toward the *Law of One—the Law of Love.*

By reconnecting with the highest vibration of love, we can begin to move forward with clarity and strength, no matter what life throws at us in the present or future. Embracing change means letting go of old patterns, especially those that no longer serve us. Holding on to past ways of living, thinking, or planning can feel safe, but in times of rapid change, clinging to outdated ideas or goals can leave us feeling out of sync. Instead, we're called to shift into a new understanding of who we are—beyond our earthly identities—remembering that we are multidimensional beings with needs that transcend the physical world.

Change does not have to be fast to be effective. Often, it is about allowing yourself to dream, to ask questions, to listen to the subtle calls of your soul. Whether change comes suddenly or gradually, it is a sign of growth, and when we trust in this process, we can move toward a more fulfilling life.

Believing in ourselves, nurturing self-confidence, and maintaining a positive self-image are key to creating miracles and laying the foundation for achieving what once seemed impossible. By thinking big, setting ambitious goals, and pushing boundaries, we can inspire ourselves to take action—and in turn, inspire others to do the same, setting off a ripple effect of growth and transformation.

Our attitude is the key to unlocking the full potential of our lives, shaping the way we perceive and respond to the world around us. Our moment-by-moment attitude shapes the reality we experience. By choosing a positive outlook and aligning with the highest vibration—*Love*—we can cultivate a mindset of success and fulfillment.

When we consciously choose to reshape our mindset, we create a foundation for a future that is limitless in possibilities.

Practice: Cultivating Inner Resilience Through Change

Change is an inevitable part of life, yet it often brings uncertainty and discomfort. When we view change as an ally rather than an obstacle, we open ourselves to growth, transformation, and the unfolding of our highest potential.

Developing resilience in the face of change allows us to navigate life's transitions with confidence, grace, and trust in the bigger picture. These practices are designed to help you connect with the energy of transformation and align with its lessons.

By grounding yourself, reflecting on past experiences, and visualizing your adaptability, you can build a foundation of inner strength that allows you to embrace the unknown with openness. Through these steps, you'll learn to see change not as a disruption but as a pathway to self-discovery and growth.

Explore these practices especially when you feel overwhelmed or uncertain. Over time, you'll notice a shift in how you approach challenges, seeing them as opportunities to expand and evolve.

Grounding in the Present Moment

Find a comfortable, quiet space. Sit or lie down, close your eyes, and take a few deep breaths. Allow yourself to settle, feeling your body supported by the earth beneath you.

Bring your awareness to your breathing, noticing each inhale and exhale. As you breathe, imagine roots extending from your body, grounding you to the earth. Feel a sense of stability, knowing that no matter what changes occur, you are rooted in the present moment.

Reflect on Past Changes

Recall a significant change or challenge from your past that ultimately led to growth or understanding. Reflect on how you felt during that time, what you learned, and how it transformed you. Ask yourself:

What strengths did I develop through this experience?

How did this change contribute to who I am today?

Writing down your reflections can be helpful, as it allows you to see patterns of resilience and growth.

Visualize Embracing Future Change

With eyes closed, visualize a future version of yourself who has fully embraced the energy of change, someone who is flexible, resilient, and open.

Picture this future self smiling and at peace, accepting change with grace and trust. Notice the qualities that you would like to embody—strength, calm, joy, adaptability, or trust. Allow this visualization to fill you with confidence.

Creating Affirmations of Openness and Resilience

Based on your reflections and visualization, create a few affirmations that resonate with your experience and goals. Some examples might be:

I welcome change as a path to growth and discovery.

I trust that life is guiding me toward my highest potential.

I am resilient, adaptable, and open to new experiences.

Repeat these affirmations to yourself daily, especially in moments of doubt or discomfort.

Set an Intention for the Week

Set a small intention for the coming week that supports your openness to change. This could be something as simple as:

I will try one new activity this week, or *I will let go of one habit that no longer serves me.*

Check in with yourself at the end of the week. Reflect on any insights, challenges, or feelings that came up as you practiced staying open to change.

Through practices like these, you begin to trust that each change is part of a larger picture, guiding you toward growth and alignment with your true self. By grounding yourself, reflecting on past lessons, and visualizing your future, you strengthen your ability to adapt to life's unpredictability with confidence and grace.

Embracing change as a friend, rather than resisting it as an enemy, allows you to transform even the most difficult moments into opportunities for growth and self-realization.

In time, this openness to change allows miracles and new possibilities to unfold naturally, leading you to the life you were meant to live. Trust that every step, no matter how challenging, is guiding you to a fuller expression of your soul's purpose.

*"Peace comes from within.
Do not seek it without."*[7]

—Budda

CHAPTER 4

FREEDOM AND HAPPINESS STEM FROM INSIDE OF US: WELCOMING YOUR INNER JOY

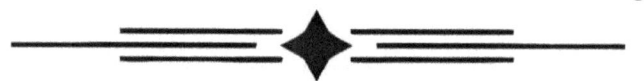

In our fast-paced, external-focused world, we often search for freedom and happiness outside of ourselves—whether through material possessions, relationships, or external achievements. However, true freedom and lasting happiness are not found in the external world but within us, in our inner essence. These qualities are always innate and available to us. We simply need to learn how to tap into them by embracing our inner joy.

Buddha's teachings on the *Four Noble Truths and the Eightfold Path* offer a path to liberation from suffering, which is often the root of our unhappiness. According to *Buddha*, true freedom comes from letting go of attachment to external desires and realizing that happiness is an inside job. The practice of mindfulness, meditation, and self-compassion are central to his teachings as ways to release suffering and experience inner peace.

We live in a society that constantly tells us that happiness is something to be attained through external circumstances. This is the illusion of external fulfillment. We are taught to chase after success, wealth, status, or approval from others as the ultimate means to feel fulfilled. But this is just a fleeting form of happiness—a temporary high that fades as soon as we achieve the next milestone.

The truth is that the pursuit of external validation often leaves us feeling empty, disconnected, and still searching for something more.

True Freedom: The Mindset of Happiness

Despite the difficulties in the world around us, some of the most fulfilled and resilient people—spiritual leaders and individuals who have endured great hardship—have found happiness and inner peace even in the face of physical deprivation or poverty. The lives of figures like *Thich Nhat Hanh, Anne Frank, Nelson Mandela, Mother Teresa, Mahatma Gandhi* and countless others stand as a powerful testament to the fact that true freedom comes not from what we possess or the circumstances we're in, but from the mindset we cultivate.

When we place our happiness in external things, we are at the mercy of circumstances beyond our control. Life's ups and downs, the actions of others, and the unpredictability of the world will always affect our mood and sense of well-being. The real source of happiness, however, lies not in the external world, but in our ability to access the joy that resides within us.

True freedom is the ability to be ourselves, without being defined by external expectations or limitations. Inner freedom comes from letting go of the beliefs, fears, and attachments that bind us. It is the liberation from the need for approval, the need for constant validation, and the need to control outcomes. When we embrace our authentic selves, free from judgment and external pressures, we experience a deep sense of peace and contentment.

True freedom and happiness come from within. We have the power to choose how we think, feel, and act in every situation. Take a moment to reflect: *What recent choices have you made that helped you rise above a challenge or experience a greater sense of freedom?* Although we may feel controlled by external events or circumstances, the truth is that their power over us is often temporary. When we take full ownership of our inner world, we reclaim our freedom and can begin to let go of the external burdens that weigh us down.

Living with Presence and Purpose

"Happiness is not something that you seek, it is something that you create from within yourself."[8] *– Sadhguru*

By learning to be present with ourselves and trusting our inner wisdom, we unlock a freedom that no external situation can give us. We no longer feel trapped by the constraints of societal expectations or by the judgments of others. Instead, we can live with a sense of ownership over our lives and our choices, confidently navigating the world in a way that aligns with our true desires and values.

Sadhguru teaches that the key to inner joy and freedom is spiritual awareness. He emphasizes the importance of taking responsibility for our inner experience and recognizing that our happiness is not dependent on the external world but on how we manage our thoughts, emotions, and energy.

The path of inner joy can be a very daunting one. Inner joy is not a fleeting emotion or a result of external circumstances—it is a state of being, a deep sense of contentment and peace that resides within us. It is the ability to find joy in the simplest moments: in nature, in creativity, in connection with others, and in the act of self-love.

To embrace our inner joy, we must first cultivate awareness of it. This means becoming present in our lives and tuning into the moments that bring us joy, no matter how small. It involves shifting our focus from what is lacking to what is abundant. Gratitude is one of the most powerful tools in this process—by acknowledging and appreciating what we have, we open ourselves to more joy.

Meditation and mindfulness practices can also help us tap into our inner joy. These practices allow us to quiet the noise of the outside world and connect with our inner selves, creating space for joy to emerge. By sitting in stillness, we give ourselves permission to simply be, without the pressure to do or achieve anything. In these moments, joy arises naturally, as we reconnect with the truth of who we are.

For many of us, fear and limiting beliefs prevent us from fully embracing our inner joy. We may fear that we are not worthy of happiness or that it is only available to certain people. We may hold onto past disappointments, mistakes, or trauma, which cloud our ability to feel joy in the present.

To experience true freedom and happiness, we must release these fears and beliefs. This process of healing and self-discovery may require introspection, self-compassion, and sometimes even therapy or counseling. By letting go of the stories we tell ourselves about who we are and what we deserve, we make room for the truth of our unlimited potential to emerge.

The Ripple Effect of Inner Joy

When we cultivate inner joy and freedom, we don't just transform our own lives—we also influence those around us. There is where it comes the ripple effect of inner joy. Joy is contagious, and by embracing our own happiness, we inspire others to do the same.

As we live with authenticity, peace, and love, we create a ripple effect that spreads throughout our communities, encouraging others to seek their own inner freedom and joy. In this way, embracing our inner joy not only leads to personal fulfillment but also contributes to a more harmonious and connected world. We can become beacons of light for others, showing them that true happiness and freedom come from within and are available to everyone who chooses to tap into their inner well-being.

Freedom and happiness are not external achievements; they are the natural states of being when we align with our true selves. By embracing our inner joy, we reclaim our power, overcome the limiting beliefs that have held us back, and create a life that is fulfilling, authentic, and abundant.

The path to inner joy begins with awareness, mindfulness, and a willingness to let go of fears and self-imposed limitations. As we unlock this source of happiness within us, we not only transform our own lives but inspire others to do the same, creating a world where joy and freedom are accessible to all.

Practice: Releasing Barriers to Inner Peace and Joy

Cultivating inner freedom and happiness begins with a conscious decision to connect with yourself and your inner resources. This is an ongoing journey of removing the mental, emotional, and energetic blocks that keep us disconnected from our natural state of being. These barriers often stem from fear, doubt, past hurts, or self-limiting beliefs that cloud our ability to embrace the present moment fully.

By intentionally creating space for reflection, mindfulness, and self-compassion, you can gently release these obstacles and reconnect with the wellspring of joy and peace within you.

These practices involve intentional moments of presence, self-reflection, and mindfulness, helping you nurture inner joy and peace.

Anchor Yourself in the Present Moment

Practice Deep Breathing: Find a quiet space to sit comfortably. Close your eyes and inhale deeply through your nose for a count of four, hold the breath for a count of four, and exhale slowly through your mouth for a count of six. Repeat this cycle for a few minutes.

Body Scan Meditation: Bring attention to different parts of your body, starting at the top of your head and slowly moving down to your toes. Notice any sensations, tension, or areas of ease, releasing tension as you go.

Embrace Joy in Simplicity

Mindful Observation: Look around your environment and pick one object or detail to focus on, such as a candle flame, a pattern, or the texture of a surface. Spend a few moments observing it closely, noticing its colors, shapes, and intricacies.

Savoring Practice: Choose an activity you enjoy, such as drinking tea, listening to music, or reading. Fully immerse yourself in the experience, paying attention to every detail, and appreciating it as though it's your first time.

Cultivate Inner Freedom Through Visualization

Imagine Your Safe Space: Close your eyes and picture a place where you feel completely at peace—a beach, a forest, or a cozy room. Visualize every detail of this place, from the sounds to the scents, and immerse yourself in its tranquility.

Freedom Visualization: Envision a situation where you feel completely free and joyful. Focus on the emotions this vision evokes, carrying those feelings into your day.

Practice Letting Go

Release Exercise: Write down any thoughts, worries, or negative emotions that weigh you down. Take a moment to reflect on them, then either shred or crumple the paper, symbolizing their release.

Mantra for Letting Go: During meditation, silently repeat a mantra such as: *I release what no longer serves me and embrace peace.*

Celebrate Small Wins

Daily Achievements Journal: At the end of each day, write down three small victories or positive moments you experienced. This reinforces a mindset of appreciation and self-empowerment.

Self-Celebration Ritual: When you achieve something, no matter how small, take a moment to acknowledge and celebrate yourself, even if it's just a smile or a happy dance.

Bring Joy into Your Routine

Create a Morning Ritual: Start your day with a practice that brings you joy, such as stretching, journaling, or listening to uplifting music.

Incorporate Playfulness: Dedicate a few minutes to something fun and spontaneous, like drawing, dancing, or trying something new.

Create a Personal Affirmation for Inner Freedom

Develop an affirmation that reminds you of your inner strength and freedom. Some examples could be:

My happiness and freedom come from within.

I have the power to choose my thoughts and responses.

I embrace the present moment and let go of worries.

Repeat this affirmation to yourself whenever you feel trapped by external circumstances, reconnecting with your inner sense of peace.

Through these practices, you begin to experience happiness and freedom that aren't dependent on external events but come from within. As you learn to pause, breathe, and embrace the moment, you tap into a source of peace that's always available to you.

Happiness and peace are always within your reach, waiting to be rediscovered.

"You are not a drop in the ocean. You are the entire ocean in a drop." [9]

—Rumi

CHAPTER 5

WE ARE A BEAM OF LIGHT: AWAKENING TO OUR DIVINE ESSENCE

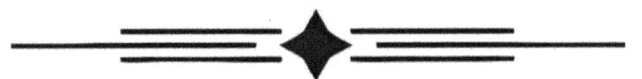

R*umi's* poetry often explores the theme of *Oneness*. His teachings remind us that we are all expressions of the divine, inseparable from the universe. Our true nature is not separate from the love and light that permeates everything; it is the essence of all existence. To awaken to this truth is to realize that the divine is not outside of us—it is within us, waiting to be recognized.

If we could perceive ourselves energetically, we would instantly recognize that we are all beams of light. I relate with the analogy that our lives are like beams of light that accumulate dust and need occasional cleansing. With this image in mind, every event in our lives can be seen as an opportunity to purify and perfect our light.

True happiness, as we learn from spiritual teachings, is not something high or external; it is deep and rooted within.

A Course in Miracles (ACIM) and *A Course of Love (ACOL)* present profound teachings on the nature of reality.

ACIM offers a clear understanding of the mind's ego-based thought system, while *ACOL* addresses the heart. In *ACOL, Jesus* speaks of uniting the mind and heart in a state he calls *"wholeheartedness,"* which leads us to a deeper understanding of oneness. Our false sense of separateness must be replaced with the truth of union—a concept best realized through our relationships with one another.

Oneness—The Interconnectedness of All Things

Everything is interconnected through *Oneness*, and all things exist in relationship. Each thing is in harmony with something else, depending on something else—nothing exists in isolation. Even the Sun, which seems to exist in the emptiness of space, is still in relationship with the vastness of space itself. *Oneness* is the undeniable truth of existence, and separation is merely an illusion.

The ego has created a false belief that we are separate from everything, but in truth, the entire universe is a beautiful dance of cooperation, where giving and receiving flow endlessly. When we align with *Oneness,* we enter a state of consciousness that flows with the universe, where we are deeply connected and fully immersed in the cycle of giving and receiving.

Jesus taught that we should not worry about our lives and pointed to the ravens, who neither sow nor reap, yet are fed by *God,* reminding us that worrying does not add a single hour to our lives. He also spoke of the lilies of the field, which neither toil nor spin, yet are clothed in splendor far greater than even *Solomon*'s finest garments. In the *Oneness* of reality, all our needs are already met.

Love encompasses everything, and nothing is left out. When we believe in our separateness, we disconnect ourselves from the unity of creation, causing us to feel that our needs are unmet. The ego focuses on perceived lack, interpreting unmet needs as evidence of deficiency.

ACIM teaches that only what we have not given can ever seem lacking. To heal the belief in lack, we must confront it, acknowledge its existence, and then release it back into the universe in some form, trusting in the flow of abundance.

The Power of Self-Love

If you are feeling lonely due to past experiences of separation, breakups, or mistreatment, it may feel like love is missing from your life. When you believe love is absent from your reality, the key is to start by giving love to yourself and radiating it outward. Go outside and connect with the love in nature, animals, children, or the people you encounter. Offer love through acts of service to others and watch how love begins to flow within and through you.

As you do this, you shift from a place of wanting to receive love to becoming a giver. You no longer seek love, recognition, or kindness from others; instead, you aim to offer these to the *Creator*, becoming the source of love. As *ACIM* teaches, giving and receiving are one and the same; what you give away is what you keep for yourself, because ultimately, you are the *Creator* in your highest form. You will only truly understand love by extending it to others.

Sometimes, we enter partnerships not with the expectation of being completed, but to realize the depth of love we already carry within. A relationship is not about seeking to get something but about recognizing that we already have everything within ourselves. In the reflection of another, we often discover the fullness of our own love.

We need to stop chasing joy and happiness and instead make our lives a true expression of them. Understand that nothing we seek externally—whether from others or circumstances—can give us lasting fulfillment. All of it originates from the *Source* within ourselves. By embracing and holding that love, and as we evolve, awaken, and journey through self-discovery, our lives naturally transform into a pure expression of *Love*, a harmonious dance of giving and receiving.

Awakening to Our Divine Essence

"When you let go of who you are, you become who you might be."[10]—*Lao Tzu*

The journey of awakening to our divine essence is not a destination, but a continuous process of growth and expansion. It requires us to be open, to question the beliefs that have shaped us, and to let go of everything that no longer serves our highest good. It is a journey of remembering who we truly are— divine beings of light, capable of infinite love and limitless potential.

Lao Tzu's teachings in the *Tao Te Ching* focus on the importance of letting go of the ego and allowing ourselves to flow with the natural rhythms of life. This aligns with the idea that awakening to our divine essence requires us to release our attachments to false beliefs and step into the flow of love, abundance, and peace.

Practice: Awakening to Our Inner Radiance Through Love and Generosity

Connecting to our inner radiance through love and generosity nurtures a sense of belonging to the world around us. It reminds us that our light is a gift, not only to ourselves but to the collective. By consciously cultivating love, sharing our unique essence, and embracing the flow of giving and receiving, we become active participants in the universal dance of light.

These practices are designed to help you connect deeply with your inner light, experience the flow of giving and receiving, and feel a sense of *Oneness* with the world around you.

Ground Yourself and Connect with Your Breath

Find a comfortable space, close your eyes, and take a few slow, deep breaths. Imagine each inhale bringing in pure, vibrant energy, and each exhale releasing any tension or negativity.

Picture a beam of light within you, starting from your heart and expanding with each breath. See this light as pure and radiant, representing your inner essence.

Visualize Giving and Receiving Love

Imagine yourself standing in a circle with all the beings around you—people, animals, plants, and the Earth itself. See each being as connected to your own beam of light, all part of the same divine source.

As you breathe, picture yourself sending love outward. With each exhale, imagine your love flowing through your light beam and touching everyone around you. As you inhale, feel the love and positive energy returning to you, creating a cycle of giving and receiving.

Embrace Wholeness: Acknowledge Your Light and *"Dust Spots"*

Reflect on any areas of your life where you may feel a sense of lack or *"dust spots"* on your light. Maybe you feel a lack of love, peace, or self-worth.

Rather than judging these feelings, embrace them as part of your human experience. Acknowledge that these are invitations to cleanse your light through acts of giving and compassion.

Radiate Love into Your Daily Actions

Throughout your day, look for ways to express this inner light and love. You might offer a kind word to a stranger, a compassionate ear to a friend, or a small act of service.

As you do this, remember that giving and receiving are one and the same. Each act of love you offer reinforces the love within you.

Affirm Your Inner Source of Happiness and Love

End the practice by repeating an affirmation that helps you internalize this truth. Here are a few examples:

I am a radiant beam of love and light, connected to all things.

My joy and love come from within, and I choose to share it freely with others.

In Oneness, I find peace and purpose, knowing I am whole.

Practice Loving Presence and Awareness in Relationships

In your relationships, remember that you don't need others to complete you; rather, you share your wholeness with them. Be aware of this in moments of connection.

Approach partnerships and friendships as opportunities to reflect and express the love that already exists within you, rather than as sources to *"get"* anything from.

These practices are meant to reinforce the idea that joy, love, and light come from within. Generosity is not simply the act of giving; it is the willingness to share from the fullness of our hearts, trusting that the more we give, the more our inner radiance grows. In turn, this light inspires others, creating ripples of joy, connection, and healing.

As you go through your days, let go of the need to pursue happiness outside of yourself. Instead, treat your life as an opportunity to express the love and light that is already within you.

By doing this, you embody the joy and freedom of being a true beam of light in the world.

*"You must be the change
you wish to see in the world."*[11]
—Mahatma Gandhi

CHAPTER 6

YOUR LIFE IS NOT HAPPENING TO YOU—IT'S HAPPENING FOR YOU: TRUST THE PROCESS

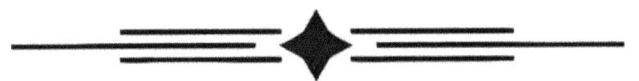

L ife is a series of lessons and experiences that, when viewed through the right lens, reveal profound opportunities for growth and transformation. The events that challenge us, our personal struggles, are not simply random occurrences but powerful tools for spiritual awakening. Once we understand this, we can shift our perspective and see that everything in our lives is happening *for* us, not *to us.*

This realization has the potential to profoundly change how we relate to the difficulties we face and to our spiritual evolution. This begins with trusting that the challenges we face are part of our personal evolution, leading us closer to our highest truth. When we experience hardship, it is easy to fall into the trap of feeling victimized or helpless. Whether it's dealing with a chronic illness, going through a divorce, enduring mistreatment, or facing betrayal, it's natural to feel like life is happening *to us.* Yet, beneath the surface of these painful experiences lies an invitation for us to learn, grow, and evolve.

Every challenge presents a lesson that, if embraced, can help us expand our consciousness and move closer to our true selves. For instance, illness may prompt us to re-evaluate our lifestyle, our approach to self-care, and our mental and emotional well-being. Betrayal may teach us about the importance of setting healthy boundaries or trusting our instincts. These experiences act as signposts, guiding us toward the next phase of our spiritual journey.

However, if we ignore the lessons hidden within these challenges, they will often resurface in different forms. Life continues to present us with the same lessons, until we take the time to integrate them.

When we truly learn from the hardships we face, we are able to transcend them and move forward with greater wisdom and insight. The lessons learned then become stepping stones toward a more enlightened and fulfilling life.

Spiritual Age vs. Physical Age

It is not uncommon to encounter individuals in their 70s or 80s who, despite their years, may still be spiritually young. These individuals might continue to face the same challenges repeatedly, not because they are *"cursed"* or unlucky, but because they have yet to fully integrate the lessons these experiences bring.

Spiritual growth isn't necessarily about the passage of time; it's about our willingness to learn from life's experiences. Spiritual maturity comes when we embrace our lessons and awaken to the deeper truths that life presents. Life continues to offer us the gift of awakening, presenting us with the same issues until we choose to learn from them.

This is a powerful reminder that spiritual growth doesn't happen automatically with age. Just as physical maturity requires effort, so does spiritual maturity. Only when we acknowledge and integrate the lessons life brings, we begin to attract the people, circumstances, and opportunities that align with our highest potential.

The Power of Self-Inquiry and Growth

As we become aware of the patterns in our lives, we gain the power to break free from them. By engaging in self-inquiry, we can reflect on what each challenge reveals about us. This process of introspection opens us to new ways of thinking, feeling, and acting, allowing us to spiritually mature and break free from cycles of repetitive experiences.

When we approach life's struggles with curiosity and openness, we cease to see ourselves as passive victims of fate. Instead, we begin to see ourselves as active participants in our spiritual evolution. Each challenge, no matter how painful, becomes an opportunity to grow, to learn, and to move closer to the truth of who we really are.

At the heart of this transformation is the realization that the *Divine, God, the Universe* is not separate from us but resides within us. This connection empowers us to see that we are not helpless beings at the mercy of fate, but co-creators of our reality. Every situation, whether joyous or painful, contains within it a divine invitation for growth, healing, and awakening.

When we embrace this perspective, we understand that life is not a series of random events, but a well-orchestrated process of spiritual growth. Even the most challenging moments are infused with divine purpose, offering us the tools we need to awaken to our true nature. As we learn to trust this divine flow, we step into a space where miracles, peace, love, and fulfillment naturally unfold.

The Path of Enlightenment and Transformation

Choosing to heal and grow spiritually means embarking on a path of enlightenment. This path is not easy, but it is always rewarding. As we integrate the lessons life brings, we move closer to our highest potential. On this journey, we become more than just the sum of our experiences. We become beings of light, guided by wisdom, compassion, and an unwavering trust in the process of life. With each step, we are led toward greater self-realization and a deeper connection to the divine source that flows through us.

The key to spiritual growth is recognizing that everything in our lives is happening for us. The challenges, the setbacks, the moments of doubt—all of these are opportunities for us to learn, to grow, and to evolve. When we embrace these lessons, we step into our power as conscious co-creators of our reality.

Life is not happening to you—it is happening for you. Each challenge, each lesson, and each moment of growth is a gift that propels you forward on your spiritual journey.

Trust in the process, and know that as you learn from each experience, you will attract the people, circumstances, and blessings that align with your highest truth. This is the path of spiritual transformation, and it is always unfolding within you.

Practice: Seeing Challenges as Spiritual Gifts

The journey of spiritual growth and self-discovery is often marked by challenges that seem difficult at first glance but are, in fact, powerful opportunities for transformation.

Through reflection, mindfulness, and intentional action, you can integrate the wisdom that comes from your experiences, heal old wounds, and break free from limiting patterns. Each practice encourages you to engage with life's challenges with trust, openness, and a deep sense of purpose, allowing you to embrace your spiritual evolution and align with the divine flow of life.

Embracing Life's Challenges as Spiritual Lessons

Reflect on Your Current Challenges: Write down the difficulties you're currently facing. For each challenge, ask: *What could this situation be teaching me about myself?*

Identify Growth Opportunities: Consider how these challenges could help you develop qualities like patience, resilience, or self-awareness.

Repeat to yourself: *This challenge is here to help me grow. I embrace it with trust and courage.*

Rewriting the Narrative of Your Struggles

Recall a Past Challenge: Think of a significant difficulty you've overcome in the past. Write about how it shaped you positively.

Shift Your Perspective: For any ongoing struggle, reframe the narrative by focusing on the lessons or strengths it's helping you build. For example, change *Why is this happening to me?* to *What is this teaching me?*

Gratitude Practice: Write down three things you're grateful for that arose from a past or current challenge.

Turning Hardship into Growth Opportunities

Self-Inquiry Exercise: Take a quiet moment and ask yourself: *What recurring patterns or situations do I notice in my life?*

Analyze the Patterns: Reflect on how these patterns might stem from unaddressed fears, beliefs, or habits.

Set an Intention: Commit to breaking free from one repeating pattern by taking a specific, intentional action. For example, if you struggle with setting boundaries, choose one area of your life to assert yourself this week.

Trusting the Divine Flow of Life

Meditation on Trust: Sit quietly for a few minutes and visualize yourself being carried by a gentle river. Imagine the river represents the flow of life, guiding you exactly where you need to be. Repeat daily: *I trust the process of life. Everything is unfolding for my highest good.*

Letting Go Ritual: Write down fears or doubts that prevent you from trusting life. Burn or tear up the paper as a symbolic act of release.

Breaking Free from Repeating Life Patterns

Awareness Exercise: Write down the challenges you've faced multiple times in your life. Reflect on what lessons you might be resisting or avoiding. For each pattern, ask: *What action can I take to break this cycle?* Commit to implementing one small change.

Visualization for Freedom: Close your eyes and imagine yourself free from the recurring struggle. Picture the kind of life and energy you'd have once the pattern is resolved.

These practices encourage reflection, self-awareness, and proactive steps toward transformation, helping you embrace life as a journey designed for your growth and highest good. By consistently incorporating these practices into your life, you can cultivate a mindset of growth, acceptance, and spiritual maturity.

The challenges you face will no longer feel like random events, but integral parts of your journey, each with its own lesson to teach. Remember, spiritual growth is a lifelong process, and with each step you take, you are deepening your connection to your true self and your highest potential.

Embrace this journey with trust, knowing that everything is happening for you, not to you.

"The primary purpose of any relationship is not to provide happiness or fulfillment, but to help you grow in awareness. "[12]

—Eckhart Tolle

CHAPTER 7

TRANSCENDING KARMIC LOVE: THE PATH TO EMOTIONAL FREEDOM

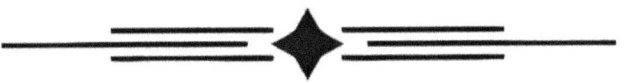

L ove is often idealized as a magical, permanent connection, but in reality, it is a profound journey filled with lessons, growth, and healing. Each relationship can be seen as an essential part of our soul's development. According to spiritual perspectives, love relationships often come with a *"soul contract"*—a pre-incarnational agreement between two souls to help each other grow and evolve.

These relationships aren't always smooth; they can be intense, revealing deep-seated issues from past lives that resurface in the present, often called *"karmic baggage."* This baggage manifests as patterns, unresolved issues, or challenges that are intended to be addressed and healed within the relationship.

In many spiritual traditions, karmic relationships are seen as opportunities to heal wounds from previous lifetimes. These relationships aren't just accidents—they are purposeful, each offering specific lessons that help us grow spiritually. They are a catalyst for this growth, teaching us to become more aware of our unconscious thoughts, behaviors, and triggers.

While some karmic relationships are relatively light, others can feel intense, sometimes triggering insecurities, fears, or unresolved emotions that need to be faced. These relationships bring lessons from past lifetimes into the present, allowing us to release the weight of old emotional wounds and break patterns that have been carried through time.

The Two Phases of Karmic Relationships

1. Initial Attraction (The *"Soul's Hook"*):

The first stage is often marked by intense attraction—an overwhelming pull between two individuals that seems to defy logic. This stage, often filled with chemistry and excitement, is driven by powerful neurotransmitters like dopamine and oxytocin. The attraction is not random; it is thought to be a *"soul's hook,"* drawing two people together so they can begin their journey of healing. This phase can feel like destiny, and many people describe it as a love that feels *"meant to be."* However, it's also a time when both individuals are often unconscious of the deeper purpose behind their connection.

2. The Reality Phase (Facing Karmic Patterns):

After the initial euphoria fades, the true work begins. In this phase, unresolved patterns and karmic baggage from both individuals' pasts begin to surface. The relationship may become rocky as emotional wounds, insecurities, and unhealed traumas come to light. This stage can be difficult because it requires both partners to face their shadows—the unconscious, suppressed parts of themselves that they've been avoiding. The challenge here is to confront these unresolved emotions and patterns, often triggering intense conflicts, but ultimately offering the opportunity to heal and grow.

Healing the Karmic Baggage Together

At the core of a karmic relationship is a mutual commitment to healing. Both individuals in a karmic relationship come into each other's lives as mirrors—showing each other where healing is needed. These relationships demand that we become more conscious, more loving, and more forgiving. The true gift of a karmic relationship is the potential to evolve together—transcending old patterns and embracing the lessons that emerge.

This perspective shifts the idea of love from a romanticized, idealized connection to a sacred partnership based on growth and transformation. In this type of relationship, both individuals are challenged to reflect deeply on their actions, words, and feelings, learning how to forgive, let go, and truly understand one another.

Setting boundaries in any relationship—whether romantic, familial, or professional—is about clearly communicating how you wish to be treated and creating a safe, respectful space for everyone involved. It's not healthy to self-sabotage or shy away from expressing the boundaries you've identified as necessary.

While these boundaries should be communicated gently and clearly, their purpose is to foster understanding and connection, not to create distance. Rather than simply drawing lines, they are meant to bring people closer together. Boundaries help reveal whether a relationship or partnership is rooted in competition or cooperation. Someone who values connection and your happiness will approach your concerns with a spirit of cooperation.

However, if your boundaries are met with defensiveness or competition, the person may prioritize their own autonomy over mutual respect, neglecting their responsibilities toward you. In contrast, a cooperative mindset prioritizes the well-being of both individuals, recognizing that only through harmony and mutual respect can a relationship truly thrive.

When one or both partners choose to grow from these lessons, a new dimension of love and harmony can be achieved.

Sometimes healing isn't always about staying together - the soul contract is fulfilled when both individuals have learned what they need to, after which they may part ways, still transformed by the journey they shared. The transformative nature of karmic love reveals and recognizes that even if the relationship ends, the growth and healing have served their purpose.

Ultimately, the purpose of karmic relationships is to transcend them. As we heal, we let go of the karmic bonds that once kept us trapped in old patterns and emotional entanglements. These relationships are not the end of the journey but a crucial part of our spiritual evolution. Through the healing of karmic baggage, we move closer to emotional freedom, allowing love to be expressed more freely, without the constraints of past hurts.

As we heal, we create space for a love that is free of past attachments, a love that is based on present, unencumbered connection and deep mutual understanding.

Practice: Healing and Growing with Your Partner

In every meaningful relationship exists a profound opportunity for growth, healing, and transformation. When we come together with a partner, we aren't just joining lives on a surface level—we're embarking on a spiritual journey that has the potential to bring us closer to our truest selves.

Within this dynamic lies the possibility for immense personal and shared evolution. This practice is designed to help you, and your partner recognize and work through karmic patterns or unresolved emotional wounds together.

Preparation

Find a quiet, comfortable space where both you and your partner can sit together without interruption. Set an intention to approach this practice with openness, vulnerability, and a spirit of mutual support.

Reflect on the Soul Contract

Start by closing your eyes, taking a few deep breaths, and setting a silent intention to connect with the deeper purpose of your relationship. Hold each other's hands and reflect on the idea that you may have come together to help each other heal, grow, and evolve. Silently ask: *What lesson is my soul here to learn through this relationship?* Each of you can take turns sharing any insights or impressions that come up.

Identify Patterns and Karmic Baggage

Consider together if there are recurring patterns in your relationship that cause conflict or tension. For example, one of you might feel abandoned or insecure, while the other struggles with expressing vulnerability.

Once identified, discuss these patterns without judgment. Approach this discussion as if you're examining something outside yourselves rather than blaming each other.

Create a Safe Space for Forgiveness and Release

Sit in silence for a few moments, focusing on the intention to let go of any past resentments or emotional blocks. If there are specific hurts or misunderstandings, take turns speaking and genuinely listening to each other, using phrases like: *I understand how you felt,* or *I forgive myself and you for the pain we both experienced.*

Allow a few moments of silence after each exchange, visualizing these issues dissolving as you release them together.

Reaffirm Your Commitment to Growth

Hold hands and take a moment to acknowledge that growth often requires patience, resilience, and continuous effort. Together, set a positive affirmation or commitment to support each other's healing, such as: *We commit to seeing each other as whole and to learning together.* Repeat this or a similar affirmation together, feeling the strength of your shared intention.

Embrace Joy and Connection

End the practice with something joyful and connecting—a dance, a shared meditation, or even just looking into each other's eyes for a few moments in silence. This can help to rekindle love and reinforce the positive energy between you.

Karmic healing within a relationship is a process, and growth occurs in stages. Continue to support each other's individual paths, honoring each person's needs and boundaries. Revisit this practice periodically to keep clearing any new patterns that emerge.

Remember that a loving, karmic relationship isn't just about romance but about partnership, mutual healing, and the shared journey toward deeper self-understanding and fulfillment. Through commitment and self-awareness, these relationships can lead to profound transformation and a more fulfilling love.

"Love is the only force capable of transforming an enemy into a friend."[13]

—Martin Luther King Jr.

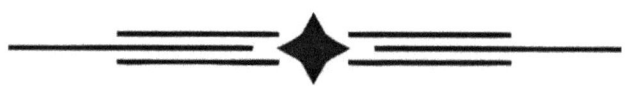

CHAPTER 8

ALL HEALING IS BASED ON LOVE: UNLOCKING THE POWER WITHIN

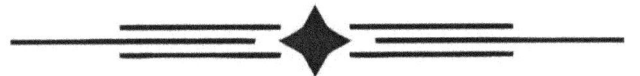

Healing is not merely about mending wounds or curing illnesses; it is a profound journey of the soul, deeply rooted in the power of love. This love is the universal force that connects us all and serves as the catalyst for transformation, not just in our bodies but also in our minds, hearts, and spirits. Understanding that all healing is based on love is the first step in aligning ourselves with our true essence and unlocking the infinite potential that resides within us.

When we consider the idea of *"healing,"* we must first recognize that love is the foundation of it all. Love is the essential energy that flows through every living being, transcending all illusions of separation and connecting us to the universe and each other.

Love heals because it restores harmony, clears blockages, and aligns us with our higher selves. It is the force that fuels our growth and guides us through the challenges of life. The more we embody love, the more we align with our true purpose, and the more healing becomes possible in all areas of our lives—whether it be our relationships, careers, or health.

Reframing Dominion from Dominance toward Responsibility

The concept of *"dominion"* over the earth, as taught in many spiritual traditions, is often misunderstood. Historically, dominion has been interpreted as dominance over the earth, leading to environmental destruction and exploitation.

A shift in perspective reveals that true dominion is about responsibility—the responsibility to nurture ourselves, each other, and all of creation. Just as a gardener nurture the seeds to help them grow, we must care for our own souls, tending to our needs with love, compassion, and patience. This practice of nurturing extends outward to others, forming a network of healing energy that connects us all.

Love is the nourishment that helps us grow and evolve into our fullest selves. Think of your soul as a seed that requires love, light, and water to sprout, grow, and bloom. Without these elements, it cannot fully realize its potential.

In this analogy, love is both the seed and the gardener, the very force that enables us to transform from a dormant potential into a flourishing reality. Life, like a garden, requires consistent nurturing. Without love, there can be no growth or self-realization.

Love and The Ripple Effect of Compassion

Healing is not a solitary act. As we heal ourselves through love, we naturally begin to heal others. This process forms a powerful ripple effect that can spread far beyond our immediate circle. When we extend compassion, kindness, and understanding to others, we activate the healing energy that circulates through all beings.

This interconnectedness reinforces the notion that love is not just an individual experience; it is a shared force that can uplift humanity as a whole. By helping others heal, we are simultaneously healing ourselves and contributing to the collective evolution of consciousness.

Love is our soul's greatest teacher, guiding us through the twists and turns of life. It teaches us patience, resilience, and self-awareness. As we awaken to the truth that all healing is based on love, we begin to see that every challenge, pain, or setback we face is an opportunity for growth. Life's difficulties are not obstacles, but lessons designed to deepen our connection with ourselves and the universe.

Each experience—whether joyous or painful—holds a lesson in love, which ultimately brings us closer to the truth of who we are. Our higher self is the part of us that is always connected to the source of all love. It is the part of us that holds the wisdom of the universe, guiding us toward our true path. When we align with our higher self, we align with love, as love is the very essence of who we are. By tapping into this deeper connection, we can navigate life's challenges with grace and ease, trusting that love will always lead us to where we need to be. Our higher self is never disconnected from us; it is always there, guiding us, loving us, and helping us remember the truth of our divine nature.

When we recognize that love is the foundation of healing, we begin to see that true healing is a collective effort. As we heal ourselves, we contribute to the healing of those around us, creating a cycle of compassion and unity. Healing through love involves recognizing our shared humanity and supporting each other on our spiritual journeys. This collective healing is not just for individuals but for all of creation, as we are all interconnected, and the health of one is impacting the health of all.

Incorporating love into every aspect of our lives
There are several ways to practice love-based healing:

Self-compassion: Treat yourself with kindness and forgiveness. Love yourself fully, accepting both your strengths and weaknesses.

Gratitude: Cultivate gratitude for the people, experiences, and lessons that life brings. Gratitude helps to align us with the energy of love and abundance.

Acts of Kindness: Extend love to others through small acts of kindness, whether it's a smile, a kind word, or a helping hand.

Meditation: Practice regular meditation to connect with your higher self and the divine love that flows through you. This practice can help you stay grounded and centered in love.

Forgiveness: Let go of grudges and resentments, as they block the flow of love. Forgiveness is essential for both personal healing and collective healing.

As we awaken to the truth that all healing is based on love, we step into our true power as co-creators of our reality. Love is the transformative force that can heal all wounds, repair broken relationships, and bring peace to our hearts.

Practice: Understanding Love as the Catalyst for Healing

When we support each other, we activate love's energy, healing not only ourselves but contributing to the healing of others and the world as a whole.

This practice is designed to help you harness love as the core energy in your healing journey. It encourages deep alignment with your higher self, compassion for others, and a sense of unity with the universe.

Preparation

Find a quiet space where you can sit comfortably and focus without distraction. Set an intention for healing—for yourself, for others, or for a specific area of life. Visualize love as a powerful light that can flow to wherever it is needed.

Self-Love Activation

Close your eyes, take a few deep breaths, and bring your attention to your heart center. Visualize a warm, radiant light within your heart. Imagine this light expanding with each breath, filling your entire being with love, compassion, and warmth.

Silently affirm: *I am worthy of love, I am filled with love, and I am healing.* Repeat this affirmation slowly and with intention, allowing it to resonate deeply.

Healing Through Unity

Extend the light in your heart outward, visualizing it connecting with the hearts of others around you—your loved ones, friends, people you've met, and even those you haven't. Imagine this network of hearts, each one connected by a thread of love, creating a web of light that surrounds the world.

Silently say: *We are all connected through love; our healing is shared.* Feel the warmth and unity within this vast connection.

Sending Love to Specific Areas of Life

Now, bring to mind any specific area where you seek healing, such as relationships, career, finances, or physical well-being. Imagine directing a beam of love from your heart to this area, enveloping it in healing light. Visualize any obstacles dissolving, leaving behind clarity, peace, and possibility.

Affirm: *Love flows freely here; healing is unfolding.* Take a few moments to sit with this image, breathing slowly, and feel the peace this brings.

Offering Love as Service to Others

Imagine how you might be able to extend love through your actions. This could be offering kindness, sharing your time, helping someone in need, or simply offering a kind word. Silently set an intention, such as: *Today, I will let love guide my actions.* When you feel ready, open your eyes and make a note of one small, specific way you'll share love with someone today.

Closing with Gratitude

Take a few moments to silently give thanks for the love within you and the opportunity to share it. Affirm: *I am grateful for the healing power of love, within and around me.* Allow this gratitude to fill you as you bring the practice to a close.

This practice can be revisited anytime you need to reconnect with love's energy or when you're seeking healing for yourself or others. Beyond meditation, let love-based intentions guide your daily actions. Small gestures like smiling, listening deeply, or offering words of encouragement help reinforce love as the foundation of your life.

When challenges arise, remember to pause and connect with the love within you before responding. Through this practice, healing becomes more than an individual journey—it becomes a shared experience of love's enduring, transformative power. And as you move forward, remember that every loving thought, word, and action you offer is an act of healing, bringing light and peace to yourself, to others, and to the world.

"Love and compassion are necessities, not luxuries. Without them, humanity cannot survive."[14]

—Dalai Lama

CHAPTER 9

EMBRACE YOUR SUPERPOWER: A JOURNEY TO UNLOCK LIMITLESS POTENTIAL

The journey to unlocking our true potential begins with recognizing the incredible superpowers we each possess, often hidden beneath layers of fear, distraction, and limiting beliefs. At the core of these superpowers lies *love*—a transformative energy that transcends all barriers and connects us to others.

Love is an incredibly powerful force, and when we embody love, we activate a superpower that has the ability to heal, uplift, and connect us with others. Love is the energy that transcends all barriers, heals wounds, and brings us into alignment with the divine. When we live from a place of love, we tap into a wellspring of wisdom and strength that can help us navigate any challenges.

This power of love is intricately linked with the practice of *mindfulness.* When we are mindful, we are fully present in each moment, allowing us to connect deeply with the essence of who we are—peaceful, centered, and grounded. It is through mindfulness that we learn to observe our thoughts and emotions without becoming entangled in them, clearing away mental clutter and returning to our true selves.

In this state of presence, we can become more attuned to the subtle beauty of the world around us, whether it's the warmth of the sunlight, the sound of birds, or the calmness of a deep breath. These moments of mindfulness help us navigate life with clarity, purpose, and a sense of calm that empowers us to act with intention.

True power also lies in the ability to *surrender*. In a world that constantly pushes us to dictate outcomes and stay in control, surrender invites us to release our need to force things and trust the natural flow of life. Surrender does not mean giving up or being passive; instead, it is an active choice to let go of resistance and trust that the universe has a plan for us.

By surrendering, we make space for new opportunities to emerge, stepping into a state of peace and faith that things are unfolding as they should. In moments of uncertainty, when we let go of worry and fear, we open ourselves up to the guidance of life's natural flow, allowing us to move through challenges with grace and patience.

Gratitude is another powerful force that shapes our experience. When we practice gratitude, we shift our focus from what we lack to what we already have, changing our perspective and raising our vibrational frequency. This simple yet profound shift allows us to see the abundance in our lives, even in the most challenging times.

By acknowledging the blessings, we have, whether it's the love of family, good health, or the beauty of nature, we align ourselves with the frequency of abundance. Gratitude not only invites more positivity into our lives but also helps us attract more of what we desire, reinforcing the belief that the universe is always providing for us.

In addition to *love, mindfulness, surrender, and gratitude, self-reflection* holds the key to unlocking our inner wisdom. By taking the time to pause and reflect on our thoughts, actions, and desires, we gain clarity and insight into our true motivations. Self-reflection helps us understand our inner truth, guiding us toward greater self-awareness and personal growth. It enables us to make more conscious choices and align our actions with our highest values and deepest desires.

Through this practice, we come to realize that everything we seek externally already exists within us, and by cultivating this inner wisdom, we are able to navigate life with greater purpose and fulfillment.

Embracing Presence and Mindfulness

A key element of being present is cultivating conscious awareness in everything you do. This practice involves becoming aware of your thoughts and how they shape your emotional and physical experiences. It's about noticing the habitual patterns of thinking that limit you and actively choosing to replace them with empowering beliefs.

For example, when a negative thought arises—whether it's a self-doubt, fear, or worry—you have the power to pause, observe it, and choose a different perspective. Instead of reacting to a stressful situation with anxiety, you can choose to approach it with calmness and clarity. Over time, you develop the ability to maintain peace and focus, no matter what external circumstances are occurring.

Similarly, your emotions are powerful messengers that tell you where you are energetically. Emotions like fear, anger, and frustration often arise from a misalignment with your true self, and they signal a need for change. By becoming aware of your emotions and the thoughts that trigger them, you can shift your internal state and take actions that align with your highest good.

For instance, if you feel overwhelmed or stuck, you can consciously choose to take a step back, breathe deeply, and refocus your energy on what is within your control.

Your actions are the outward expression of your inner world. They are the physical manifestation of your mindset, beliefs, and emotions. By consciously choosing actions that align with your goals and intentions, you reinforce the empowered mindset that you are building. This creates momentum, where each positive action you take builds upon the last, leading to even greater achievements and deeper alignment with your superpower.

Awakening to Your True Potential

"Imagination is everything. It is the preview of life's coming attractions."[15] *- Albert Einstein*

We all have unique superpowers that are waiting to be awakened. These superpowers are not just abstract concepts but practical tools that help us navigate the complexities of life with grace and wisdom.

By embodying these qualities, we step into our true potential and create a life that is aligned with our highest self. This journey of awakening is not an end goal, but an ongoing process of growth, transformation, and self-discovery—one that is driven by the power of love and guided by the wisdom within us. When we awaken to our superpowers, we unlock the ability to create, heal, and transform not only our own lives but also the world around us.

The key is to believe in our potential, embrace our inner power, and continuously strive to awaken to the fullness of who we are. The universe is ready to respond to the energy we radiate. It's time to step into your superpower and live your most extraordinary life.

Practice: Unlock the Limitless Potential Within

Being *"awake"* to our potential is about cultivating an empowered mindset and embracing life as a conscious creator. It is a process of tapping into the infinite resources and possibilities that lie within us, realizing that we are not merely passive recipients of life's experiences but active participants in shaping our destiny.

Here are some strategies and daily practices to help you align with your most awakened self, tapping into states of consciousness where clarity, purpose, and intuitive insight thrive.

Set an Empowering Word of the Day

Start each morning by choosing a word that represents the energy or focus you want to embody that day. Words like *clarity, love, alignment, strength*, or *courage* can set a powerful tone.

As you go about your day, reflect on this word. Visualize yourself embodying this quality and watch how this practice shifts your actions and mindset.

The Silva Method for Problem Solving

Developed by *José Silva,* this technique teaches you to enter a relaxed, meditative Alpha state to resolve problems and attract synchronicities.

Before Bed: Identify a specific issue or goal. As you fall asleep, focus on a solution or positive outcome, setting the intention for insight to come to you. Begin with deep breathing to relax and slowly count down from 100 to 1. With practice over 30 days, you'll decrease the countdown, eventually reaching an Alpha state within seconds. This helps *"program"* your mind to relax and receive insights.

In the Morning: Reflect on any new ideas or synchronicities that might relate to your problem. Often, insights come through subtle *"aha"* moments or as clarity in your thoughts.

Visualize Your Ideal Day as a Creator

Each morning, take a few minutes to visualize your day unfolding in alignment with your intentions. Imagine yourself moving through the day with grace, strength, and purpose. Envision challenges as opportunities and visualize yourself responding calmly and effectively.

As you imagine your day, hold a feeling of gratitude and excitement, allowing this positive energy to set the tone.

Edison's Theta Technique for Inspiration

Edison used a creative technique to access the Theta brain state—associated with intuition and creativity—by relaxing to the point just before sleep.

Sit comfortably, close your eyes, and hold a small object in your hand (like a pen or ball). As you relax deeply, focus on any area where you seek inspiration. Allow yourself to drift into relaxation. If you start to lose the object as you doze, gently wake yourself and note any ideas or images that come to mind. Over time, this practice helps you access the Theta state more easily, unlocking creative insights.

Journaling and Reflection

Daily Self-Check-In: Write down what it means to you to be *"awake"* today. Reflect on any doubts or beliefs that might limit you. Challenge these thoughts by rewriting them in a positive light.

End-of-Day Reflection: Spend a few moments each evening reviewing your day. *How did you align with your intentions? Did your empowering word guide your actions?* Recognize any small victories or moments of growth.

Setting Larger Goals: Each month, choose a theme or personal quality to focus on (such as *strength*, *compassion*, *wisdom*, or *confidence*). Journal about how you want to develop this quality and break it into smaller, achievable steps you can focus on daily.

Accessing Delta States for Transformation

Delta is a deep, restful brainwave state where profound healing and transformative change can occur. Typically achieved in deep sleep or very deep meditation, it can help *you "program"* positive changes into your subconscious. While Alpha waves are occurring in a relaxed and aware state, to achieve Delta waves requires different level of awareness, typically and primarily present during deep sleep. As well, Theta waves are achieved at the point just before sleep.

At night, after reaching the Alpha state through relaxation techniques (such as counting down), affirm a phrase connected to your personal power, like: *I am infinitely capable, and every day I awaken closer to my true potential.*

Over time, this nightly affirmation may integrate into your subconscious mind, helping you naturally shift toward growth-oriented thoughts and actions.

Living Your Highest Potential: A Mindset of Self-Awareness

Cultivate Awareness: Recognize moments when you're on *"auto-pilot."* When you catch yourself, gently bring your focus back to your goals and values.

Practice Kindness: Approach all relationships from a place of kindness and openness, measuring others by the goodness in your heart rather than reacting to negativity.

Celebrate Progress: Each small step counts. When you experience synchronicities, personal growth, or breakthroughs, take time to celebrate. Gratitude and acknowledgment fuel your motivation.

By following these practices and exploring new ways of thinking and being, you can begin to connect more deeply with your own *"superpower"* and potential. Awakening to your limitless potential is not an end goal; it's a daily, evolving practice that will continue to shape the best version of you. Embrace this journey with patience, openness, and excitement, knowing that the life you envision is always within reach.

"You are infinite. You have the ability to be anything, and you are only limited by your own thoughts."[16]
—*Dolores Cannon*

CHAPTER 10

COMING HOME TO THE INFINITE YOU: UNLOCKING THE TRUTH OF WHO YOU ARE

D*olores Cannon* words hold a powerful truth: the only limits we have are the ones we place upon ourselves. Our potential is boundless, waiting to be unlocked by the awakening of our inner power. The most profound way we can honor ourselves and others is by embracing our fullest potential every day. When we shift from a mindset of limitation to one of possibility, we begin to experience life as conscious creators, shaping our world with clarity, purpose, and intentionality. The journey of awakening to our true selves is transformative, offering endless opportunities for growth, creativity, and empowerment.

In a world that often pulls us in different directions, it is easy to lose sight of who we truly are. We can become tangled in the past, in fears, and in societal expectations, all of which obscure the deep connection to our authentic selves. However, there comes a time when we are called to come back home—to reconnect with the infinite being within us, to embrace our power, and to step fully into our divine purpose.

Coming home to the infinite you is about remembering who you truly are—an infinite being capable of boundless love, creativity, and wisdom. It is about aligning with the essence of your soul, living with intention, and bringing light into the world around you.

It is safe to let go of old wounds, regrets, and fears that no longer serve you. Often, we cling to the past out of comfort or habit, but this only holds us back from stepping into the fullness of our power. The moment we release the past, we create space for the present moment, and the present moment is where our true power resides.

By trusting that life is unfolding as it should, we can stop fearing the future and begin to take inspired actions that align with our soul's purpose.

Aligning with Your Soul's Purpose

"Our deepest fear is not that we are inadequate. Our deepest fear is that we are powerful beyond measure."[17]*- Marianne Williamson*

Living in alignment with your soul's purpose is not a passive endeavor. It requires conscious awareness and a commitment to living authentically. It means stepping into the truth of who you are, beyond the roles and expectations imposed by society. Many of us fear our own greatness, our own potential, but this fear is rooted in false beliefs. When we let go of this fear and trust that we are here to make a positive impact, we unlock the full force of our potential. However, in order to fully embrace this experience, we must also take responsibility for our lives and actions. We are creators, and it is through our choices that we shape our reality.

Sometimes, this means stepping out of our comfort zones and embracing our superpowers. We must shift our mindset from *"I can't"* to *"I can."*

We are capable of far more than we often realize, and by believing in our own power, we unlock the door to a life of limitless possibilities. We owe it to ourselves and our future selves to live in alignment with our soul's purpose and to take inspired action in every moment.

It is about letting go of the past, trusting in the flow of life, and stepping into your purpose with love, mindfulness, and courage, embracing the light within and letting it shine out into the world. As you align with your soul's purpose and trust in the divine process, you will see that everything you need is already within you. Trust yourself, trust the process, and embrace the infinite potential that awaits you. Your time is now, and the world is waiting for you to step into your power and shine.

When you truly believe that you are capable of extraordinary things, you begin to see life as a canvas full of possibilities. Your belief in yourself creates an invisible force that attracts the people, resources, and opportunities necessary for your growth. This belief transforms ordinary moments into extraordinary experiences, turning obstacles into stepping stones on your journey of self-discovery.

Reconnecting with Your True Essence

The essence of who you are—your authentic self—is not something you must create or find; it is already within you, waiting to be rediscovered. Your being is powerful beyond measure, capable of love, wisdom, and boundless creativity. It is not limited by the constraints of the past or the fears of the future. It exists in the present moment, where your true power lies.

When you reconnect with your true self, you stop looking outside of yourself for answers. Instead, you begin to trust the wisdom of your soul. Spiritual leaders, philosophers, and teachers from various traditions have long spoken of the boundless potential of the human spirit. They have shared practices that allow us to tap into this infinite power and transform our lives. As you awaken to your true nature, you realize that you hold the key to the life you envision.

There is no limit to the love, wisdom, or potential that lies within you. When you come home to this truth, you tap into the deepest source of power and creativity in the universe. You begin to see the world not as a place of limitations but as a field of endless opportunities.

Living with Intention and Authenticity

One of the most transformative tools is the power of intention. Your thoughts shape your reality, and the energy you invest in them determines the direction of your life. When you set a clear intention—whether it's for healing, abundance, peace, or love—you align your energy with that desire. This is not just about thinking positive thoughts but about embodying the energy of what you wish to create. For instance, if you desire to cultivate more compassion, you begin by setting the intention to be compassionate in every interaction, allowing that energy to flow freely through you.

In doing so, you not only manifest more compassion in your life but also become a beacon of light for others, guiding them toward their own healing and growth. This is the power of living with intention: you create the life you seek by embodying the truth of who you are.

At the heart of coming home to the infinite you is the decision to live authentically. This means stepping away from the roles, labels, and expectations placed upon you by society. It is about embracing your true self and living in a way that reflects your soul's deepest desires. By doing so, you unlock your unique gifts, and the world becomes your canvas to create a life full of meaning and purpose.

By walking this path of self-discovery, you become a beacon of hope, love, and possibility, lighting the way for others to come home to the infinite truth of who they are. This is a transformative journey of awakening and self-discovery.

As you release the past, embrace the present, and trust in the divine flow of life, you unlock your infinite potential. The life you desire is already within you—it is waiting for you to claim it.

Practice: Letting your true self guide your actions

Your inner self—the core of who you truly are—holds the wisdom and clarity needed to navigate life's challenges and opportunities. It is when you connect with your authentic self that you begin to align with your soul's purpose and move through the world with ease and confidence.

Embracing the infinite you is a transformative journey that requires daily practices to nurture and awaken the full potential within you. This journey is not about reaching a destination; it is a continuous unfolding of your soul's highest expression.

The following practices guide you toward living a life of authenticity, love, and empowerment—becoming the conscious creator of your reality.

Living with Intention

Living in alignment with your soul means understanding your deepest desires, values, and calling. To tap into this purpose, take moments to reflect, listen to your inner guidance, and let your soul lead the way.

Soul Connection Ritual

Each morning, set an intention to connect with your higher self. Acknowledge that you are more than your current situation and that your soul holds the wisdom of the universe. Sit quietly and ask yourself: *What does my soul want to express today? How can I bring more light into my interactions?*

Visualize your day unfolding with purpose, filled with opportunities for love, connection, and growth. Trust that everything will align when you respond intuitively from your soul's guidance.

Embracing Divine Timing

Trusting in divine timing is a key part of your journey. The universe operates on its own schedule, and part of your growth is learning to trust that what is meant for you will come when the time is right. Whenever impatience or frustration arises, pause, and remind yourself that the life is never in a rush. Everything is unfolding in its perfect timing.

Practice gratitude for the present moment. Reflect on all the blessings you currently have and recognize how they align with your soul's growth. Trust that more is coming in alignment with your highest good. Keep a journal to track moments of synchronicity or unexpected blessings as a reminder that divine timing is at work.

Shifting Your Mindset

Your infinite potential lies in your mindset, creativity, and ability to bring light into dark situations. Changing limiting beliefs is key to unlocking your power.

Whenever you face self-doubt, ask yourself: *What if I could? What would I do if I believed in my unlimited potential?*

Shift from a *"I can't"* mindset to a *"I can"* mindset by choosing a small action that aligns with your dream. Even a tiny step is progress. Use affirmations like:

I am capable of achieving great things.

I trust in my power to create a positive impact.

I am a unique force of love and light.

Embracing Your Autonomy and Power

Your autonomy is your power. By taking control of your life and decisions, you create space for your highest self to emerge and fully express itself. Every time you face a decision, ask yourself: *Does this choice align with my soul's purpose? Am I acting from a place of love and authenticity?*

Cultivate awareness in each moment. Remember that you are the creator of your life. By taking responsibility for your thoughts, feelings, and actions, you reclaim your autonomy.

Celebrate every step you take toward self-empowerment. Reflect on how your actions shape the life you desire and bring you closer to your divine essence.

Finding Joy in the Journey

The journey of awakening is meant to be joyful. Don't get so caught up in reaching a specific destination that you forget to enjoy the process. Embrace moments of joy and play. Life is meant to be fully experienced, with laughter, love, and lightness. Engage in activities that make you feel alive—whether it's dancing, creating, or spending time with loved ones.

Let go of the need for perfection. Trust that as you move with the flow of life, everything will fall into place. Embrace each moment as it comes.

These practices encourage you to live in the moment, fully experiencing life's joys while navigating the ups and downs with grace. As you embrace your true essence, you become the conscious creator of your life's unfolding.

When you let your true self guide your actions, you embrace the wisdom and power that have always been within you.

By trusting this inner compass, you move through life with clarity and purpose, knowing that each step you take is an authentic expression of who you truly are. When you act from this place of alignment, you not only come home to the infinite you, but you also become a radiant beacon for others to follow.

"There are seven planes of being...
each plane is an ascending scale of vibration,
from the lowest to the highest."[18]
— *Helena Blavatsky*

CHAPTER 11

THE SEVEN DENSITIES: A PATH OF EVOLUTION AND CONSCIOUSNESS EXPANSION

The concept of the *Seven Densities* provides a profound framework for understanding the evolution of consciousness and its progression through various states of awareness. This model offers an intricate map of spiritual development, correlating with the chakra system, where each density represents a higher level of consciousness, each one a stepping stone toward unity and enlightenment.

These densities reflect the shifting energies and frequencies of both individual beings and the universe at large, showcasing how consciousness evolves over vast spans of time.

The First Density: The Root Chakra (Red)

The journey begins in the first density, corresponding to the *Root Chakra*. This stage marks the initiation of consciousness in its most elementary form. At this level, consciousness interacts with the five basic elements—earth, water, fire, air, and space—shaping the material world. It is a time of raw existence, where consciousness is focused on survival and the foundational forces that drive the development of physical life.

In the context of this density, the experience is primitive and focused on grounding, where life is crystallized through geological processes and environmental forces.

The Second Density: The Sacral Chakra (Orange)

The second density represents the realm of growth and movement. Here, consciousness expands beyond mere survival and begins to express itself through more complex forms of life, such as plants, animals, and microorganisms. This stage is associated with the *Sacral Chakra*, a center of vitality and creativity.

The key feature of this density is the development of life that is dynamic, evolving, and capable of movement. Consciousness at this stage begins to embody the concept of growth and change, adapting to its environment and learning to interact with other living beings.

The Third Density: The Solar Plexus Chakra (Yellow)

The third density is often referred to as the *Density of Separation.* It is the level of human consciousness, where the experience of individuality and separation from others becomes prominent. This density corresponds to the *Solar Plexus Chakra*, which governs personal power, ego, and self-esteem.

In this density, humans experience duality, the tension between the positive and negative aspects of existence. It is within this separation that both the potential for great good and the capacity for harmful actions arise. They are not inherently evil but are often unaware of the deeper, universal truth of oneness, resulting in actions motivated by fear, ego, and a desire to assert control.

The Fourth Density: The Heart Chakra (Green)

The fourth density marks a significant transformation, as consciousness begins to transcend the illusion of separation. It is the realm where love and oneness emerge as the fundamental truths of existence. This density corresponds to the *Heart Chakra*, the center of compassion, connection, and unity.

In the fourth density, individuals start to embrace love as the core of their reality, understanding that they are interconnected with all beings. This shift is essential for transcending the suffering and conflict that arise in the third density and is crucial for moving beyond the limited perspective of individual separation.

The Fifth Density: The Throat Chakra (Blue)

The fifth density is where wisdom, light, and expression come to the forefront. This density aligns with the *Throat Chakra*, which governs communication and truth. As consciousness ascends to this level, it becomes more refined, and the ability to express deeper truths about existence is unlocked.

In the fifth density, beings understand the universal laws that govern reality, and they use their communication to share wisdom and guide others on their spiritual paths. This density represents a time of clarity, where the soul begins to integrate its understanding of the world and to express itself in higher vibrational ways.

The Sixth Density: The Third Eye Chakra (Indigo)

The sixth density represents the ultimate balance between love and wisdom. It is a stage where consciousness has evolved to a point where both the heart and the mind are harmoniously integrated. This density corresponds to the *Third Eye Chakra*, the center of intuition, insight, and higher consciousness. At this level, souls are fully aware of the interconnectedness of all life and understand that all actions, thoughts, and beings are part of a greater whole.

The consciousness in the sixth density operates with profound wisdom and compassion, navigating the complexities of existence with a deep understanding of the universe's mysteries.

The Seventh Density: The Crown Chakra (Violet)

The seventh density is the highest level of consciousness in this model, representing the culmination of spiritual evolution. It is the stage where consciousness fully realizes its oneness with the universe. This density corresponds to the *Crown Chakra*, the center of divine connection and enlightenment.

Beings in the seventh density are no longer bound by physical form, existing instead as pure light and electromagnetic energy. They embody the ultimate truth of unity, having transcended all duality and realized the infinite nature of consciousness. In this state, beings are completely integrated with the universal source, understanding that all life is interconnected, and that separation is an illusion.

The Path of Service: Positive and Negative Polarity

As consciousness progresses through the densities, it faces a choice between two primary paths: service to others and service to self. These paths represent opposite approaches to growth and spiritual evolution.

Service to Others (Positive Path): This path focuses on selflessness, compassion, and the well-being of all. Those who walk this path seek to transcend their ego and operate from a place of love, recognizing that their true nature is intertwined with the collective consciousness. The positive path ultimately leads to the realization of oneness and the dissolution of the illusion of separation.

Service to Self (Negative Path): The negative path, in contrast, is centered around control, fear, and selfishness. It is a path of domination and manipulation, where beings attempt to separate themselves from others to gain power. However, this path ultimately leads to a paradox, as the being reaches a point where it can no longer grow or evolve. The negative path forces individuals to confront the truth of oneness and often leads to a reversal of polarity, pushing them toward the positive path.

The Journey of Ascension

"The heart is like a polished mirror, reflecting the Divine truth. As we polish it, it reflects more light."[19] *— Rumi*

The journey through the seven densities represents the spiritual evolution of consciousness, where each density corresponds to a higher level of awareness, from the basic survival instincts of the first density to the enlightened unity of the seventh.

As consciousness ascends, it sheds the illusion of separation and moves toward the realization that love, wisdom, and unity are the ultimate truths of the universe.

The path of ascension is a gradual process of spiritual refinement, where beings evolve through cycles of learning and growth. This journey is not just a personal transformation but a reflection of the larger, cosmic process of evolution, where all of existence moves toward greater understanding and unity.

The *Seven Densities* offer a powerful lens through which we can view our own spiritual development, guiding us toward higher consciousness and the realization that *Oneness* is the highest truth of the universe.

Practice: Seven Densities of Awareness as Evolutionary Blueprint

The seven densities of awareness provide a profound evolutionary blueprint for understanding the spiritual journey of consciousness. Much like the chakras represent stages of energetic alignment, these densities outline the cosmic path of growth, where individuals and collective beings expand in awareness and vibration.

Each density corresponds to a distinct phase of development, from the elemental foundations of existence to the ultimate realization of unity with all creation.

Through this framework, you can explore how consciousness progresses through survival, self-awareness, love, wisdom, and unity, ultimately transcending duality to embrace oneness with the universe. This blueprint serves as a guide for personal transformation, inviting you to align with the higher frequencies of love, wisdom, and service.

The following practices are tailored to help you resonate with the lessons of each density and support our spiritual evolution.

First Density: Root Chakra (Red)

This is the density of survival, corresponding to the Root Chakra, where consciousness begins to crystallize. At this stage, consciousness interacts with the elements—earth, water, fire, air, and space—gaining knowledge through the fundamental forces of nature.

Ground yourself daily by connecting with nature, walking barefoot, or meditating while focusing on stability and survival. Practice mindful breathing and affirmations to connect with the earth's energy.

Second Density: Sacral Chakra (Orange)

This is the realm of growth, movement, and vitality, associated with plants, animals, and microorganisms. Consciousness in this density develops the ability to grow and move through the physical world.

Engage in creative activities, such as dancing, drawing, or gardening, that encourage vitality and growth. Open your heart to the life force within nature and explore your passions to expand your creative expression.

Third Density: Solar Plexus Chakra (Yellow)

The third density is the realm of human consciousness, often referred to as the *"Density of Separation."* This stage is associated with the Solar Plexus Chakra, which governs personal power, self-esteem, and the ego. It is where duality and the experience of separation arise. Focus on self-love, confidence, and creating healthy personal boundaries. Reflect on your experiences of separation and work to transcend them by fostering compassion and unity with others.

Fourth Density: Heart Chakra (Green)

The fourth density represents the transition to unity, where love and oneness become the focus. This corresponds to the Heart Chakra, where compassion, empathy, and connection to others are central. It is the density of transformation, where we begin to embrace love as the core of reality.

Cultivate compassion by meditating on the heart center. Engage in acts of kindness, practice gratitude, and visualize yourself as a part of the interconnected whole. Focus on healing relationships and fostering unity.

Fifth Density: Throat Chakra (Blue)

In the fifth density, consciousness becomes more refined and expresses itself through wisdom and light. This corresponds to the Throat Chakra, which governs communication, truth, and self-expression. In this density, beings begin to understand deeper universal truths.

Work on clear and honest communication, both with yourself and others. Reflect on areas where you need to express your truth and cultivate a deeper understanding of the world. Speak with love and wisdom in your interactions.

Sixth Density: Third Eye Chakra (Indigo)

The sixth density is about balancing love and wisdom. Corresponding to the Third Eye Chakra, this density is about insight, intuition, and higher consciousness. Souls in this density have a deep understanding of the interconnectedness of all life. Engage in practices that develop your intuition, such as meditation, mindfulness, and inner reflection. Seek to balance love with wisdom and deepen your understanding of the mysteries of existence.

Seventh Density: Crown Chakra (Violet)

The seventh density represents the highest level of consciousness, corresponding to the Crown Chakra. This density is where oneness and divine connection are fully realized. Beings in this density are pure light and exist in harmony with the universe, transcending physical limitations. Dedicate time to deep meditation and reflection on your connection to the divine. Practice recognizing the interconnectedness of all life and feel the unity of all beings.

Holistic Practices for Ascension

To ascend through these densities and evolve spiritually, the following practices can support you in aligning with the higher frequencies of love, wisdom, and unity:

Daily Meditation

Dedicate time each day to meditate, focusing on each chakra in turn. Start with grounding in the Root Chakra and progress upward to the Crown Chakra, imagining each energy center glowing with light. Use visualization to connect with each density's lessons and attributes.

Practice Service to Others

Look for opportunities to help others in your life, whether through acts of kindness, volunteering, or simply listening to someone in need. Focus on service to others as a means of transcending the ego and cultivating the positive polarity.

Balance Love and Wisdom

Reflect regularly on your life to ensure you are balancing love (Heart Chakra) and wisdom (Throat and Third Eye Chakras). Seek harmony between your heart's desires and the wisdom you gain through experience. Incorporate acts of service and kindness while maintaining discernment and wisdom.

Self-Awareness

Regularly reflect on your thoughts and actions. Ask yourself whether your behavior stems from love and service or from fear and separation. Work on overcoming negative patterns and expanding your awareness of oneness.

Seek Higher Consciousness

Continue to seek higher states of awareness through study, reflection, and connection with higher beings. This can be done through reading spiritual texts, meditating on universal truths, or connecting with guides or mentors who can help expand your understanding.

Transcend the Negative Polarity

Recognize and transcend the negative aspects of yourself and the world. Focus on shifting away from fear, selfishness, and separation, and move toward love, service, and oneness. Remember, the negative path eventually reaches a paradox, leading to the recognition of oneness, which can result in a polarity shift.

Integrating More Light

As you move through the densities, work on raising your vibration and embodying more light. Visualize yourself as a being of light, integrating more of the higher frequencies available in the fifth, sixth, and seventh densities. Allow your physical and energetic bodies to align with the higher dimensions of consciousness.

The Evolutionary Blueprint of the *Seven Densities* offers a comprehensive map for spiritual growth. By aligning with the lessons of each density, you can navigate the cosmic path from survival to self-awareness, from love to wisdom, and ultimately to the realization of oneness with all creation.

Through dedicated practice, it can be transcended the limitations of separation, embodying the higher frequencies of unity, and aligning with the divine purpose of existence.

As you ascend through the densities, you will awaken to the profound truth that we are not separate beings but integral parts of a vast, interconnected whole—a journey of love, wisdom, and infinite light.

"Out of darkness, light is born."[20]

—*Lao Tzu*

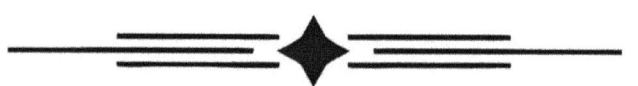

CHAPTER 12

UNITY IN DUALITY: THE PATH TO SPIRITUAL AWAKENING

The quest for understanding the nature of existence, consciousness, and the universe has occupied humanity for millennia. Various spiritual traditions and philosophies have attempted to explain the origin and purpose of life, often emphasizing the interplay between opposing forces—light and darkness, good and evil, creation and destruction.

One of the most profound teachings on this topic comes from the *Law of One,* a channeled material received in the 1980s. The *Law of One,* delivered through the entity known as *Ra,* offers deep insights into the spiritual evolution of humanity, the nature of the *Creator,* and the role of dualities in the universe. This philosophy teaches us that embracing both light and darkness is essential for growth, integration, and ultimately, spiritual ascension.

At the heart of the *Law of One* lies a fundamental truth: all of creation is one. The universe, as vast and diverse as it may appear, is a single, unified consciousness. From the smallest atoms to the farthest galaxies, everything is interconnected. This teaching challenges us to look beyond separateness and to recognize the divine unity that underlies all existence. We are not isolated beings; rather, we are expressions of a single *Source* or *Creator.*

This understanding offers a profound sense of interconnectedness with all beings. It calls for a deep awareness of our actions, thoughts, and intentions, knowing that they impact the whole of creation. In this framework, our lives are not merely a series of random events but part of a greater, divine plan that binds us all. We are not separate from others; we are one with all that exists.

Reincarnation and the Veil of Forgetting

The journey of the soul unfolds over many lifetimes and reincarnation plays a pivotal role in our spiritual evolution. Each soul's journey involves learning and growth through experience, and with every lifetime, a soul moves closer to the ultimate goal of unity with the *Creator.*

As mentioned in a previous chapter, a key aspect of this journey is the veil of forgetting—a divine mechanism that causes us to forget our past lives during our current incarnation.

This veil serves a crucial purpose: it allows us to experience each life as a new opportunity for growth and discovery without being weighed down by the baggage of previous lives. It is only upon ascending to higher densities (the fourth density and beyond) that the soul regains full awareness of its past experiences. This process of spiritual evolution becomes a quest for remembering—remembering who we truly are, reconnecting with the *Creator*, and realizing the unity that pervades all of existence.

Every soul's journey involves a choice between two primary paths of spiritual evolution: the *Path of Light* and the *Path of Darkness.*

The Path of Light is aligned with the positive polarity and is focused on service to others. Souls who walk this path prioritize the welfare of others, seeking to uplift and support those around them. They act selflessly, not from a place of personal gain, but out of a deep understanding that helping others is tantamount to helping oneself. On this path, love, compassion, empathy, and cooperation are central to one's existence.

The *Path of Darkness* is aligned with the negative polarity, which is focused on service to self. Souls on this path seek personal power, control, and dominance over others. Their actions are driven by a desire for self-interest and material gain, often at the expense of others. The negative polarity is not inherently *"evil,"* but rather a necessary force within the universe to create the contrast and challenges that catalyze growth in consciousness.

The Universal Role of Both Polarity Paths

What is most important to understand in the *Law of One* teachings is that both paths are essential for spiritual evolution. Without darkness, there would be no light. Without the challenges and obstacles created by the negative polarity, there would be no impetus for souls to seek the light.

Just as a seed needs darkness to grow and sprout into the light of day, consciousness requires the experience of dualities to catalyze its expansion. The *Creator* is not judgmental of either polarity, is the *Source* of both light and darkness. In fact, the *Creator*'s journey involves exploring both polarities in order to fully understand and experience itself.

The light represents the true nature of the *Creator*—love, unity, and creation—while the darkness represents the absence of that light, serving as a contrast through which the light becomes meaningful.

This concept is revolutionary in its implications: darkness is not the opposite of light in a dualistic sense but a complementary force that allows for the expression of the light. The *Creator* does not label the negative polarity as bad or undesirable, for it is through this polarity that the consciousness comes to know itself. The darkness exists only as a catalyst for the light, allowing consciousness to expand and deepen.

The unfolding of existence involves the manifestation of both creation and destruction, birth and death, light and dark. The negative polarity, in this sense, serves as the absence of the *Creator*'s full light, and it exists only to give context and meaning to the positive polarity. Without this balance of opposites, creation would not be able to unfold in the dynamic way that it does.

The Journey Toward Integration

"The wound is the place where the Light enters you."[21] *– Rumi*
The ultimate goal of the spiritual journey is integration. Spiritual evolution is a path of synthesis—where we integrate both the light and the dark within ourselves. Initially, we must experience both polarities to understand our true nature and to facilitate growth. However, as we mature on our spiritual path, the objective becomes to move toward the light.

This integration process involves accepting the shadow aspects of ourselves, acknowledging the darkness, and using these experiences as opportunities for growth and self-awareness. By embracing both light and dark, we achieve wholeness, understanding that the shadow is not to be feared but integrated into the greater whole.

This is where true spiritual evolution takes place: in the integration of opposites, where the soul transcends duality and aligns with the unity of the *Creator.*

Balance is crucial in the journey of spiritual evolution. As we move toward the light, we must understand that both polarities are valid, necessary, and ultimately lead to the same end goal: reunion with the *Creator.* The darkness does not need to be eradicated; it simply needs to be understood and transcended.

By embracing the dualities of creation, we align with the natural rhythms of the universe and move towards a state of spiritual harmony. The journey is not about rejecting the darkness but about understanding its role in our growth.

As we integrate these forces within ourselves, we move closer to the ultimate goal: the realization of our oneness with the *Creator* and the understanding of the infinite love that underlies all existence.

The path to spiritual evolution is not linear but cyclical, an eternal dance between light and darkness, where both play essential roles in our journey toward self-realization and unity with the divine.

Practice: The Dance of Light and Darkness

In the vast tapestry of existence, duality shapes our experiences. Light and darkness, creation and destruction, service to self and service to others—these polarities are not opposites to be fought against but complementary forces guiding our growth.

The teachings of the *Law of One* remind us that true spiritual awakening comes from integrating both polarities within ourselves. By embracing the interplay between light and dark, we transcend judgment and align with the unity that connects us to the Creator.

The following practices are designed to help you explore, accept, and integrate these dualities, fostering balance, awareness, and a deeper sense of connection with the infinite unity of existence.

Shadow Acknowledgment Ritual

Sit in a quiet space with a journal. Reflect on recent situations where you felt fear, anger, jealousy, or judgment. Write about the thoughts or behaviors that arose during those moments without judgment. Say aloud: *I see you, and I accept you as part of my journey. You are here to teach me, and I honor the lessons you bring.*

Conclude with gratitude for the insights gained from these shadows.

Light Activation Meditation

Sit comfortably and close your eyes. Visualize a golden light radiating from your heart center. With each breath, allow this light to grow, filling your entire body and extending outward to the world around you. Affirm silently: *I am a vessel of light and love, connected to all that is.*

Rest in this awareness for a few minutes, feeling the unity and wholeness of your being.

Polarity Reflection Exercise

At the end of each day, reflect on your choices and interactions. Identify actions that were rooted in self-interest and those in service to others. Ask: *How did each serve my growth or the growth of others?*

Write one intention for the next day to balance these polarities, such as offering kindness or setting a healthy boundary.

Duality Visualization

Close your eyes and imagine standing between two powerful forces: a radiant sun representing light and a vast starry sky representing darkness. Feel both energies flowing into you, balancing your body and mind. Say silently: *I am both the light and the shadow, unified in the Creator's love.*

Rest in this balanced state for a few minutes before gently opening your eyes.

Service Alignment Practice

Identify one meaningful way to support someone each week, such as listening deeply, offering help, or sharing wisdom. Perform this act with no expectation of reward, recognizing that service to others is an expression of service to yourself and the *Creator.*

The journey toward spiritual awakening is not about rejecting the darkness or clinging solely to the light—it is about embracing both as essential aspects of the *Creator's* infinite love. By integrating the dualities within ourselves, we transcend the illusion of separation and align with the unity that binds all existence.

Through these practices, you cultivate balance, self-awareness, and compassion for all aspects of your being. This integration allows you to step fully into your true nature, radiating harmony and oneness in all that you do.

As you walk the path of Unity in Duality, you become a living expression of the *Creator's* eternal dance between light and darkness, embodying the infinite potential of love and creation.

"Mindfulness is the aware, balanced acceptance of the present experience. It isn't more complicated than that."[22]

— Jon Kabat-Zinn

CHAPTER 13

THE RESCUER'S JOURNEY: EMBRACING SELF-CARE AND EMPOWERMENT

For those who embody the role of a rescuer—those who feel a deep calling to help others—there is often a point in the journey where the well-being of the rescuer becomes neglected. Caregivers, healers, and helpers may find themselves overwhelmed by their desire to serve, giving endlessly without replenishing their own energy. This imbalance can lead to burnout, resentment, and a sense of depletion.

The desire to rescue or fix others often stems from deep empathy, a genuine desire to alleviate suffering. However, without proper self-care, this impulse can lead to burnout. The rescuers may find themselves caught in a cycle of over giving, where their own emotional, physical, or spiritual needs are ignored. The healing they offer others may leave them empty, unable to restore their own vitality.

The first step in rescuing the rescuer is recognizing the need for self-care. When a rescuer begins to turn inward, they can start the healing process within themselves. Self-care is not a selfish act; rather, it is a vital practice that replenishes their energy, restores their sense of purpose, and renews their commitment to service.

By setting boundaries, acknowledging their needs, and seeking their own healing, the rescuer shifts from being a savior to an empowered being who can help others without depleting themselves.

A key aspect of this transformation is embracing vulnerability. Rescuers often carry the belief that they must always be strong for others, but true strength comes from acknowledging one's own weaknesses and caring for them. In doing so, the rescuer not only heals themselves but becomes an even greater source of strength for others.

Balancing Compassion and Self-Love

The empowered rescuer understands that helping others does not require self-sacrifice, but rather a balance between compassion for others and self-love. This shift allows the rescuer to act from a place of abundance, rather than scarcity. They recognize that their ability to offer love and care is dependent on their own emotional, mental, and spiritual well-being. They know how to set boundaries—whether physical, emotional, or energetic—so that they can maintain their own health and well-being while still serving others. They understand that they cannot pour from an empty cup, and they must first care for themselves before they can give to others.

Self-care practices such as meditation, journaling, and connecting with nature help the rescuer replenish their energy, ensuring they can continue to serve from a place of fullness rather than emptiness.

Compassion begins within. Empowered rescuers cultivate self-compassion, forgiving themselves when they falter, and offering themselves the same love and care they give to others. They understand that their worth is not tied to what they do for others, but to who they are as a divine being.

Embracing Your Role as the Host of God

Being the host of *God* is a sacred and transformative journey. It requires us to live with intention, mindfulness, and deep love for ourselves and others. By honoring our bodies as temples, cultivating presence, and caring for our own needs as rescuers, we align with our divine purpose. When we recognize that we are vessels for divine energy, we treat ourselves with reverence and care, offering our highest selves to the world.

We are all called to be the host of *God,* to be mindful of the divine presence within us, and to live from a place of empowerment and compassion. By embracing these practices and perspectives, we can create a life of profound love, peace, and service, ultimately becoming beacons of light for those around us.

Just as a host welcomes a guest into their home and offers them the best of what they have, we should nurture our bodies, minds, and souls to honor the divine presence within. This mindset of being the host of *God* is not just a fleeting thought— it is a practice, a continuous journey of living with love, intention, and mindfulness. As we cultivate awareness of our inner divinity, we become more attuned to our highest potential, embodying love and light in every moment.

In many spiritual traditions, the body is considered a temple—a sacred space that houses the soul. When you embrace the idea that your body is a temple of *God,* you begin to treat it with the reverence it deserves.

This means nurturing it with nutritious food, exercise, rest, and self-care. The mind and spirit are deeply connected to the physical body, and the care we give to our bodies directly impacts our mental and emotional well-being. To honor the body as a temple, we must also engage in mindful movement—

yoga, stretching, walking, or any physical practice that helps us stay connected to our body's energy. Similarly, rest is an integral part of honoring the body. A well-rested body creates a clear mind and an open heart, ready to serve the world with love.

By slowing down and paying attention to the needs of the body, we offer ourselves the gift of vitality, enabling us to align with our highest potential.

Cultivating Stillness and Awareness

Being the host of *God* means living with intention and presence. The practice of mindfulness—being fully present in each moment—grounds us in the here and now, allowing us to offer our full attention to whatever we are doing.

By engaging in practices that create stillness, we begin to deepen our connection to our true essence. Whether through breathwork or mindful observation, these moments of pause create space for divine wisdom to flow through us, guiding our thoughts, words, and actions. In today's fast-paced world, where doing is often prioritized over being, it is easy to forget the power of presence.

We should try to make present moment, the *NOW*, the primary focus of our life. When we take a moment to simply breathe, to focus on the present moment, we allow ourselves to reconnect one more time with the divine.

Practice: Empowering the Rescuer Within

Empowering the rescuer within requires developing a balanced approach to caregiving, where self-awareness and self-care are as prioritized as the care you extend to others.

Below are practices to guide you on the journey to self-empowerment and transformation, ensuring you can continue to offer your support to others from a place of abundance and not depletion.

Acknowledge Your Own Needs

Start by recognizing that, as a human being, you have needs too. Rescuers often forget to prioritize themselves in their quest to care for others. The practice here is to pause and reflect on your own emotional, physical, and spiritual needs. Journaling can help you identify areas of your life that need attention. Ask yourself:

What do I need emotionally, physically, and spiritually right now?

Are there areas of my life where I feel drained or unfulfilled?

How can I nurture myself to restore balance?

By acknowledging your needs, you begin the process of validating your own humanity and cultivating self-compassion.

Set Boundaries with Compassion

Setting healthy boundaries is vital to maintaining your well-being. As a rescuer, saying *"no"* can be difficult, but it's necessary to avoid burnout and empower both yourself and others. Here's how to practice boundary-setting:

Pause before responding: When someone asks for help, check in with yourself first. Do you have the energy to help them? Is this an opportunity for them to solve their own problems and grow?

Set boundaries with kindness: Saying *"no"* can be done compassionately. For example: *I understand your need, but I'm unable to help right now. I encourage you to explore other support options.*

By practicing this, you will not only protect your energy but also model healthy boundaries for those you care for.

Nurture Yourself with Love and Care

Nurturing yourself is not selfish; it's a divine act of self-love. Begin to recognize your own worth and treat yourself with the same care and compassion you give others. Here's how to practice self-care in all aspects:

Physical Care: Nourish your body with healthy food, exercise, and rest. Consider your body as a temple that requires love and maintenance.

Emotional Care: Practice speaking kindly to yourself. Forgive your mistakes and allow yourself to feel without judgment.

Spiritual Care: Meditate, pray, or connect with nature to nourish your spirit. These practices help you reconnect with your higher self and sense of purpose.

Turn Inward with Intention

As a rescuer, you may have been so focused on others that you've neglected your inner world. To shift this pattern, begin turning inward to confront your own emotional needs and unresolved pain:

Meditation and Reflection: Take time to sit in silence. Focus on your breath and allow your thoughts and emotions to come and go naturally. Ask yourself: *What parts of me need healing? What am I avoiding?*

Seek Professional Support: If needed, talk to a therapist, counselor or spiritual healer to help you work through deeper emotional blocks and to nurture your inner self.

This process of turning inward helps you grow emotionally and strengthens your ability to empower others from a place of wholeness.

Embrace the Role of Empowerment, Not Rescuing

To truly empower yourself and others, shift from rescuing to empowering. This means:

Support don't save: Rather than solving someone else's problems, encourage them to find their own solutions. Ask questions like: *What do you think would be helpful in this situation?*

Model self-love and empowerment: Show others that healing comes from within by practicing self-care, setting boundaries, and living with purpose. In doing so, you create a space for both you and others to grow and heal.

To be the rescuer you truly want to be—someone who empowers and supports others—you must first honor and nurture yourself.

By practicing self-care, setting boundaries, turning inward for healing, and embracing your role as a divine host, you not only heal yourself but become a stronger, more empowered source of support for others. When you nurture your body, mind, and spirit with love, mindfulness, and compassion, you become a beacon of light and empowerment—both for yourself and for the world around you.

"Silence is not the absence of something. It is the presence of everything."[23]

—Eckhart Tolle

CHAPTER 14

SACRED SILENCE: A GATEWAY TO INNER PEACE AND SPIRITUAL GROWTH

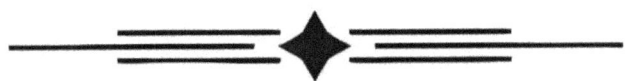

In a world overflowing with noise—both external and internal—the practice of silence offers a sanctuary for the soul. Sacred silence is more than just the absence of sound; it is a deliberate act of stepping away from life's noise and embrace stillness instead. It is within this quietude that we often discover the deepest aspects of our being, fostering spiritual growth, personal transformation, and profound inner peace.

Silence has long been revered in spiritual traditions as a pathway to enlightenment and connection with the divine. From the meditative practices of Buddhism to the contemplative silence of Christian monasticism, the power of quietude transcends cultural and religious boundaries. Silence invites us to turn inward, confronting the restless thoughts and emotions that often dominate our consciousness.

In this inward journey, we begin to unravel the layers of our conditioned mind. The distractions of daily life—constant notifications, conversations, and responsibilities—create a mental fog that disconnects us from our true selves. Sacred silence cuts through this noise, offering a clear space to reflect, reconnect, and realign with our higher purpose.

The Benefits of Silence for Spiritual Growth

The practice of silence nurtures spiritual growth in several profound ways:

Deepening Self-Awareness

When we quiet our minds, we create space for self-reflection. Silence enables us to observe our thoughts, patterns, and emotions without judgment. This heightened awareness allows us to identify limiting beliefs, unhelpful habits, and unresolved inner conflicts.

Strengthening Intuition

In the stillness of silence, we can attune ourselves to our inner wisdom. The intuitive voice, often drowned out by mental chatter, becomes clearer and more accessible. This guidance helps us make decisions aligned with our spiritual path and personal growth.

Enhancing Connection to the Divine

Many spiritual seekers describe moments of silence as opportunities to feel a profound connection to the divine or universal consciousness. In these moments, the ego dissolves, and we experience a sense of unity with all that is.

Healing and Transformation

Silence provides a nurturing space for healing. Emotional wounds, stress, and trauma often surface during silent reflection, allowing us to acknowledge and release them. This transformative process fosters inner peace and resilience.

In the absence of distractions, we connect more deeply with the essence of life and our true selves. Silence opens the gateway to inner peace and presence, allowing us to move beyond the noise of the mind and experience the stillness that is our natural state.

Practicing silence and detoxing from constant media exposure offers a profound reset that can help us reconnect with ourselves on a deeper level. By committing to even a single day of silence or media fasting, you open up space for reflection and awareness that is often overshadowed by the noise and demands of daily life.

Engaging with nature, getting quality sleep, hydrating well, eating mindfully, and grounding yourself with sunlight and earth are all simple yet powerful acts that help recalibrate your mind and body. Techniques like dark room retreats, where sensory input is limited, heighten this connection further by allowing you to focus solely on the inner workings of your mind. This extended silence reveals both the noise and depth within, eventually leading to a quieter mind and a more peaceful heart.

Such practices help reveal how layers of conditioning—formed by society, media, and even our closest influences—shape much of what we believe. Over time, these influences accumulate and take root, but practices like silence and mindful self-care peel them back, bringing you closer to your authentic self.

The more you connect with this true nature, the greater your sense of healing and the stronger your motivation to pursue personal growth and raise your inner vibration.

Creating a Daily Silence Routine

Even a few minutes of silence each day can be transformative. Begin each morning or end each night in silence, taking time to simply sit with yourself. Over time, this practice of daily silence becomes a refuge, a moment to reconnect, reflect, and reset.

In your silence, practice visualizing what you are grateful for. Picture the faces of loved ones, recall happy moments, or imagine nature scenes that bring you peace. Gratitude can act as a powerful tool to shift your mental state, opening your heart and mind to positive vibrations.

During your silent retreat, try fasting or eating simple, nourishing foods in small portions. Not only does this lighten your body, but it also clarifies the mind. When eating, do so slowly, savoring every bite. This practice of conscious eating becomes a form of gratitude and brings a deeper awareness of your relationship with food.

Take moments to intentionally connect with natural elements. Feel the warmth of sunlight, the grounding energy of the earth beneath your feet, the freshness of a cool breeze, or the sensation of water on your skin. These sensory experiences, even in small amounts, can help you feel more in tune with nature and with yourself.

Journaling can be an effective practice to accompany your silence. Without speaking, allow your thoughts to flow onto paper. Write without judgment—just observe your thoughts, emotions, and insights as they arise. This practice can help bring clarity to subconscious patterns and beliefs.

The Impact of Silence on Your Inner Landscape

"Silence is a source of great strength." [24]*– Mahatma Gandhi*

Silence offers a retreat from the tumult of the world, providing the strength necessary to act with clarity, compassion, and truth. By cultivating silence, you clear away the mental *"noise"* and gain insight into the layers of conditioning, beliefs, and external influences that shape you.

This process helps us rediscover who we are beneath these layers—bringing us closer to a place of inner peace, alignment, and higher consciousness. Each moment of silence is a chance to listen to the *"true self,"* the one that exists beyond labels, roles, and attachments.

In a world that constantly demands attention, silence offers a revolutionary act of self-preservation and self-awareness. Through it, we're reminded that the power of transformation lies within, waiting for us to notice. The more we embrace silence, the more we realize it's not an absence of sound but a presence—an opening to our truest selves.

Practice: The Silent Path to Spiritual Awakening

Silence, when embraced as a deliberate and sacred practice, can transform our emotional, mental, and spiritual well-being. It's not just the absence of sound; silence offers a profound presence that fosters healing, clarity, and connection with our inner truth.

Below are practices to incorporate silence into your daily life, promoting peace, growth, and spiritual alignment.

Begin Each Day with a Silent Morning Ritual

Start your day with silence to connect with your inner self. Upon waking, avoid distractions like phones. Spend a few minutes in silence, focusing on your breath or a simple affirmation: *I am grounded in peace and clarity.*

Take a Midday Silence Break

Pause for a few minutes during your busy day to reset and regain focus. Find a quiet space, close your eyes, and observe the sensations in your body. Shift your attention inward, letting your thoughts settle.

Silent Eating Meditation

Eat one meal in complete silence, free from distractions like phones or TV. Focus on the textures, colors, and flavors of your food. Chew slowly and express gratitude for the nourishment.

Create a Sacred Silence Space

Designate a small, calming area in your home for silence.

Add peaceful elements like candles, plants, or meaningful objects. Use this space daily to meditate, pray, or simply sit in stillness.

End Your Day in Quiet Reflection

Dedicate the last moments of your day to quiet self-reflection.

Turn off devices 30 minutes before bed. Write in a journal, observing your thoughts or expressing gratitude.

Engage in a Silent Nature Walk

Take a walk in nature, such as in a park or forest, in complete silence. Pay attention to the natural sounds around you and the sensations in your body. Use the walk to ground yourself and connect with the present moment.

Practice a Weekly Digital Detox

Set aside one day or evening each week to disconnect from screens. Replace screen time with silent activities like reading, journaling, or meditating. Reflect on how being away from technology impacts your peace and clarity.

Visualize Silence as Healing Energy

During moments of silence, use visualization to deepen inner peace. Imagine a soothing light surrounding you, dissolving tension and worry. Let this light fill you with warmth, stillness, and serenity.

Commit to Extended Silent Retreats

Plan a half-day or full-day silent retreat for deeper introspection. Use this time for meditation, journaling, or quiet activities. Embrace solitude as a chance to connect with your higher self.

Use Silence as a Daily Check-In

Pause for 2 minutes during the day to check in with yourself. Ask: *What am I feeling right now? What do I need in this moment?*

Use the silence to listen to your answers and guide your next steps.

The transformative power of silence strips away distractions and brings you closer to your essence and purpose. As you integrate these practices, silence will not only be a break from the world—it will become an invitation to rediscover the essence of who you truly are.

"When you change the way you look at things, the things you look at change. "[25]

— *Wayne Dyer*

CHAPTER 15

A LETTER TO MY YOUNGER SELF: A JOURNEY OF SELF-DISCOVERY AND HEALING

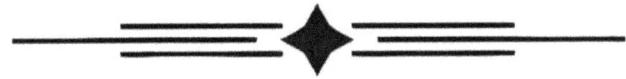

Writing a letter to your younger self can be a deeply therapeutic and transformative experience, offering an opportunity for reflection and healing. It's an exercise that can help you navigate life's challenges with more wisdom, understanding, and compassion.

By shifting how you perceive situations, you can uncover hidden opportunities and lessons within our challenges. It reminds us that our reality is not just shaped by external events but by how we interpret and respond to them. By writing to your younger self, you can change the view of past struggles—recognizing them not as obstacles but as opportunities for growth, transformation, and enlightenment.

In moments of struggle, it's often easy to feel overwhelmed. This exercise encourages you to step back and see your life from a broader, more detached perspective—as if watching a movie. You may recognize in this way that some of the hardest moments you've faced were precisely the ones that shaped you, helping you grow into who you are today. They were not setbacks but lessons that guided you toward your highest potential. We all carry a long list of struggles, pains, and heartbreaks, moments that seem insurmountable at the time. But when we step back and look at them from a distance, we can begin to appreciate their role in our journey.

These experiences are the very ones that have built our resilience, shaped our character, and provided the wisdom that now resides within us. They are not to be feared or resented but honored as the great teachers they truly are. Every challenge has had its purpose in helping us discover our strength and uncover the deeper truths about who we are.

The Role of Failure in Shaping Our Path

Failure, often seen as a setback, is an inevitable part of the journey to success. It is a necessary teacher, showing us where we need to grow, adapt, and learn. Failure is never final, and it is never a roadblock. Instead, it is simply another step on the path to personal evolution.

Through these experiences, you will learn to refine yourself, developing the qualities and mindset needed to move forward. The key to overcoming difficulties lies not in dwelling on problems but in focusing on solutions. By maintaining a positive attitude, you allow to be guided toward the right behavior and outcomes that will serve your highest good.

Integrating the Lessons—The Ongoing Journey of Self-Discovery

As you reflect on our journey, it's important to take the time to integrate the lessons you've learned. Every hardship and every triumph have brought you closer to understanding yourself and the world around you. You are here to learn and evolve, and the process of self-discovery is ongoing. By staying open to these lessons and embracing your inner wisdom, you will unlock the potential for greater success, not in the material sense, but in the sense of emotional and spiritual fulfillment.

A key component of this journey is finding the light within. No matter what life throws our way, we always carry within us the ability to shine brightly. You must continue to nurture your inner light, let go of what no longer serves you, and step into the fullness of who you are meant to be. This means embracing gratitude for everything you have in the present moment and fostering a mindset of generosity.

When we give to others—whether through love, kindness, or service—we amplify our own happiness and fulfillment.

These two practices, gratitude, and generosity can transform your experience and elevate your life to a higher vibration.

The Path to Christ-Consciousness

In *A Course of Love* we are reminded that we are living in a time of spiritual awakening. The course teaches that we are moving toward a higher state of consciousness—*Christ-consciousness*—a state of deep connection with our true selves and with others. The teachings in *A Course of Love (ACOL)* complement those of *A Course in Miracles (ACIM),* continuing the journey of integrating mind and heart into a unified state of being.

The ultimate message is that we have the potential to experience heaven on earth during our lifetime, and this can only be achieved when we live in harmony with one another, free from struggle and effort.

The beauty of this journey is that it is not about endless striving or forcing outcomes. Life, as we are meant to experience it is peaceful, effortless, and abundant. The more we align with the energy of love, the more we discover that life's challenges are not obstacles but opportunities to grow, heal, and awaken. As we journey toward self-discovery, we find that each step brings us closer to the truth of who we are—radiant beings of love, light, and infinite potential.

This letter to our younger selves is not just an exercise in reflection; it is a powerful tool for healing. By embracing the lessons of the past, integrating them into our present, and choosing to live with love and gratitude, we transform our lives. We move beyond the limiting beliefs and fears of the past and step into the full expression of who we are meant to be—whole, loving, and free.

Embracing Self-Love on Our Journey

In this journey, we realize that we are not alone. We are part of a greater whole, and through our relationships and connections, we discover the depth of our own divinity. We are all here to learn, to grow, and to evolve. As we do so, we create a more harmonious, loving world for ourselves and those around us.

We are meant to live in unity with each other, embracing the truth of who we are, and experiencing the fullness of love in every moment. As we continue our journey, may we always remember to trust the process, honor the lessons, and, above all, love ourselves deeply.

Practice: Writing a Letter to Your Younger Self for Reflection and Growth

This exercise allows you to reframe past experiences as valuable lessons, connect with your inner light, and embrace the mindset of gratitude and generosity. By writing a letter to your younger self, you create an opportunity to reframe past experiences with love, understanding, and gratitude.

It is a powerful tool for healing, enabling you to acknowledge the challenges you faced while recognizing them as valuable lessons that contributed to your growth.

This practice isn't about rehashing pain or regret but about embracing the past as a stepping stone toward the wholeness you're now capable of embodying. It allows you to forgive, honor, and celebrate who you were and who you are becoming.

Create a Sacred, Quiet Space

Find a quiet place where you won't be interrupted. Set the mood by lighting a candle, playing soft music, or having a favorite comfort item nearby. Take a few deep breaths, close your eyes, and center yourself in the present moment. Let go of any distractions and imagine connecting with your inner light.

Visualize Your Younger Self

Picture yourself at a specific younger age or during a time when you faced a significant challenge. Try to imagine what you looked like, how you felt, and the thoughts that occupied your mind. Hold compassion in your heart for this younger version of you, who was doing the best they could with the knowledge and resources they had at that time.

Begin Writing Your Letter

Start with a warm greeting to your younger self. You might say: *Dear [Your Name]*, or *Hello, Younger Me.* Write as though you are having a loving, compassionate conversation with a friend. Reflect on the challenges you know this younger version of you will face but reassure them that each one is a stepping stone, guiding them to become the person you are today.

Share Lessons Learned

Share some of the biggest lessons you've learned from your journey so far. Be gentle, encouraging, and forgiving. Mention how each struggle brought wisdom, resilience, or a new perspective. For example: *I know things feel overwhelming now, but you'll find strength in these hard times that will later help you navigate life's ups and downs.*

Emphasize Gratitude and Generosity

Express gratitude for all that your younger self has done to bring you to this point. Acknowledge their resilience, bravery, and ability to grow through adversity. Encourage your younger self to practice generosity, giving love, and kindness without expectation. Remind them that true fulfillment comes from a heart that gives freely.

Reflect on the Future with Hope and Vision

Instill a vision of hope, encouraging your younger self to trust the journey and embrace Christ-consciousness. Mention how your experiences are guiding you toward a peaceful and fulfilling life. You might include a passage inspired by *A Course of Love* such as: *You are here to experience peace and love, and to connect with the world in union. Let this journey be one of ease and joy.*

Conclude with Words of Self-Love and Empowerment

Close the letter with a few words of love and encouragement. Tell your younger self to carry these words forward, especially in moments of doubt: *You are loved. You are worthy. You are powerful. Everything you need is already within you.* End the letter with a loving closing, such as: *With love and gratitude,* or *Forever in your corner.*

Reflect and Integrate

Take a few moments to read the letter you've written. Feel the healing energy of compassion and love that this exercise brings.

Consider placing this letter somewhere special or reading it whenever you need to reconnect with your inner wisdom and strength.

To extend this practice, begin each morning with this affirmation: *I am whole, loved, and deeply connected with the flow of life. I embrace each moment with love and gratitude, radiating joy and peace in every experience.*

Throughout your day, remind yourself that you are a beam of light, here to bring love, peace, and kindness to the world. Let your life be an effortless expression of your inner truth, and trust that you are living in alignment with a higher purpose.

This practice can help you move through each day with a renewed sense of purpose, calm, and generosity, knowing that every moment is part of your journey toward peace and wholeness.

"Only when we are brave enough to explore the darkness will we discover the infinite power of our light. "[26]

—Brené Brown

CHAPTER 16

THE ANGEL WE FORGOT ABOUT: FINDING LIGHT IN OUR DARKEST MOMENTS

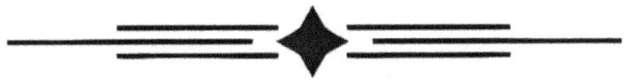

L ife is a journey filled with twists and turns, and inevitably, we all encounter moments that feel impossibly dark. These times can leave us feeling isolated, overwhelmed, and trapped in an endless cycle of pain or despair. In such moments, we often look downward, lost in the darkness, trying to solve the issue from the same level of consciousness that created it. What we forget, however, is that there's always an angel nearby—a guiding presence, a higher frequency, a lifeline—waiting to lead us out of the shadows.

The concept of *"the angel we forgot about"* is a powerful metaphor for the unseen or overlooked forces of love, grace, and guidance that are always available to us, even when we can't perceive them.

Angels don't always come in the form of winged beings from a higher plane; they can be the friend who calls at just the right moment, the quiet wisdom of a book, the stillness of nature, a song played on the radio, or the gentle whisper of our intuition. They are the reminders of a greater force at work, urging us to climb out of our despair and into a higher state of being.

The Trap of Wrestling with the Darkness

In moments of deep suffering, our tendency is to fixate on the problem. We replay the story of our pain, trying to control or resolve it at the level of the issue. But the solution isn't found in wrestling with the darkness—it's found in reaching for the light.

The angel we forgot about is the bridge, offering us a way to rise above the storm and see things from a clearer, more expansive perspective. Angels are always around us, offering their presence and guidance, if only we are willing to see and accept them.

Angels come in many forms. Sometimes they appear as loved ones who support us unconditionally. Other times, they are found in habits or practices that connect us to our higher selves—like journaling, meditating, or taking a walk in nature. They might even show up as strangers, offering a kind word or gesture that shifts our perspective. These angels are reminders that we are never alone, even in our darkest hours.

Recognizing these angels requires a shift in focus. When we are trapped in a cycle of fear or pain, our attention narrows, and we become blind to the lifelines around us. It takes courage to lift our gaze, to stop wrestling with the problem and instead reach for something higher. This act of reaching isn't about denying the darkness—it's about choosing to see the light that exists alongside it.

Each of us has the ability to connect with these angels and rise above our challenges. It begins with awareness—pausing in the midst of our struggle to ask: *What higher guidance is available to me right now?* The answer might come as a memory of someone who can help, an urge to create or express, or simply a sense of peace that allows us to take the next step.

Those guiding forces that offer love, grace, and support are not always external; they also reflect our inner strength and resilience. Understanding the dual nature of these angels—both internal and external—can help us navigate through life's challenges with greater clarity and hope.

The Angel Within and Our Own Inner Strength

These angels are not just an external force; it's also a reflection of our own inner strength and divinity. By reconnecting with this part of ourselves, we align with a higher frequency that transforms our pain into purpose, our fear into faith, and our despair into hope.

In the end, the journey through darkness is not about erasing the hardships but about discovering the light within and around us.

These angels remind us that we are never without support, even when life feels unbearable. By opening ourselves to these guiding forces—whether they come in the form of a person, a practice, or a moment of stillness—we reclaim our power and step into a higher state of being. They are both an external force and a reflection of our own inner strength. By acknowledging and embracing both aspects, we can find the light in our darkest moments and emerge stronger and more resilient.

The next time you find yourself overwhelmed by life's challenges, pause and look for the angel you may have forgotten. Whether it's a call to a friend, a moment in nature, or the quiet strength of your own heart, there is always a lifeline waiting for you to grab hold. And as you climb higher, you'll find that the very darkness that once held you down was the catalyst for your greatest awakening.

Practice: Connecting with the Angels Within and Around Us

Life's challenges can feel isolating, yet within and around us are ever-present sources of light, guidance, and strength—our *"angels."* These angels, both external and internal, act as lifelines, gently leading us toward clarity, hope, and transformation.

The following practices are designed to help you connect with these guiding forces, whether they manifest as loved ones, moments of grace, or your own inner strength. By intentionally engaging with these practices, you'll cultivate awareness, embrace resilience, and find the light in your darkest moments.

Practices to Recognize and Embrace External Angels
Gratitude Reflection

At the end of each day, list three moments when you felt supported or uplifted. These could be a kind word, a gesture from a stranger, or even a moment in nature. This practice helps you recognize the subtle presence of angels in your daily life, shifting your focus from challenges to blessings.

Angel in Disguise Exercise

Think of someone who has been unexpectedly helpful or present in your life. Write a letter (even if you don't send it) expressing gratitude for their role as a guiding force. Acknowledging these *"angels"* strengthens your awareness of external support systems.

Connecting with Nature

Spend time in nature—walk in a park, sit by water, or simply observe the sky. Reflect on how nature's beauty and stillness provide guidance and peace. Nature serves as an angelic reminder of life's cycles and the ever-present opportunities for renewal.

Community Involvement

Engage in community activities or volunteer work. Helping others can often reveal the angels in your community and create a network of mutual support. Being part of a community fosters a sense of belonging and highlights the collective strength and kindness around you

Practices to Awaken the Inner Angel

Guided Self-Compassion Meditation

Sit quietly, close your eyes, and repeat affirmations like:

I am strong. I am supported. I am capable of rising above this.

Visualize yourself surrounded by a warm light of your own

making. This meditation connects you to your inner strength, reminding you of your inherent ability to navigate challenges.

Journaling for Higher Guidance

Write down a specific challenge you're facing. Then, ask yourself: *What would my wisest, most loving self say to me right now?* Write down the response without overthinking. This practice taps into your intuition, which acts as an inner angel, offering clarity and encouragement.

Resilience Building Through Visualization

Visualize yourself overcoming a current obstacle. Imagine the steps you'll take, the support you'll receive, and how you'll feel on the other side. By visualizing your own success, you activate your inner angel of resilience and create a roadmap for action.

Practices to Integrate the External and Internal Angels

Mindful Acts of Kindness

Each day, perform a simple act of kindness—whether for a loved one, a stranger, or yourself. Be fully present as you give this kindness and notice its impact. Acts of kindness connect you with external angels and strengthen your internal sense of purpose and compassion.

Sacred Pause Practice

When you feel overwhelmed, pause for a moment. Take three deep breaths, and silently ask: *What support is available to me right now?* Be open to the answer—whether it comes as a thought, memory, or sensation. This practice creates space for both external and internal angels to guide you in times of need.

By weaving these practices into your daily life, you create a bridge to the angels you may have overlooked—the guiding forces that come in many forms. They remind us that we are never alone.

As you nurture this connection, you'll find not only the courage to face life's challenges but also the wisdom to transform them into opportunities for growth. The angel you forgot about is always waiting—ready to guide you toward your greatest awakening. All it takes is a moment of awareness to rediscover its light.

"We don't see things how they are,

we see things how we are."[27]

—Anaïs Nin

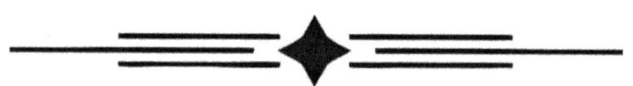

CHAPTER 17

THE LENS OF THE MIND: HOW THOUGHTS SHAPE OUR PERCEPTION OF REALITY

There is a deeper truth about lies within the very fabric of our reality. Our perception of the world is not a direct reflection of the external world but is filtered through the lens of our thoughts, beliefs, and emotions. Every individual experiences reality through their unique mental framework, and this internal lens shapes how we interpret, respond to, and engage with the world around us.

Our minds, much like a receiver, are constantly tuning into a vast collective energy field of thoughts, impressions, and experiences. In this way, our ideas, intuitions, and inspirations are not solely our own creation. Rather, they are part of a larger universal flow of energy—ideas, thoughts, and emotions that we pick up from the collective consciousness. Our thoughts are not personal, but rather they are energy forms that we tap into, becoming part of the greater web of existence.

However, just as there are positive and uplifting thoughts that inspire growth, there are also negative and hostile energies that, if not carefully observed, can become trapped in our minds. These negative thoughts can create a cycle of self-doubt, fear, and internal conflict. The more we identify with these thoughts, the more they become ingrained in our consciousness, shaping our reality and our actions.

Repetition of these negative thoughts leads to their entrenchment in our minds, making it harder to break free from them. Over time, these thoughts take on the quality of energy entities—hostile forces within the mind that attack our peace and well-being. As we begin to identify with these thoughts, we fall deeper into the trap of ego—the belief that we are these thoughts and that they define who we are.

The Practice of Becoming the Observer of Thoughts

What if we could step back and observe these thoughts instead of identifying with them? The freedom we seek lies in this very practice. The more we detach from the thought forms that arise in our minds, the more we come to realize that we are not our thoughts. We are the awareness behind them.

Thoughts are temporary, fleeting, and subject to change. They come and go like clouds passing through the sky, and only when we stop attaching ourselves to them do we begin to reclaim our true nature.

This awareness is the key to shifting our perception of reality. If we allow ourselves to become caught up in negative thought patterns, we will perceive the world as negative. If our minds are clouded with self-criticism or doubt, we will attract experiences that confirm these beliefs, reinforcing the cycle of negativity.

However, if we can shift our awareness and consciousness to a higher state, we begin to see the world not as a reflection of fear and separation but as a reflection of possibility, growth, and peace. The hidden costs of our thoughts and actions are often overlooked.

For instance, many of us indulge in distractions like social media, Netflix, or sugary drinks without realizing that they cost more than just our money. They cost us our time, our health, and our focus. Similarly, indulging in negative thought patterns costs us our peace of mind, our happiness, and our connection to the present moment. It seems more like when something is free more then likely we are the product. By investing in negativity, we become prisoners of our own minds, trapped in a cycle of suffering that we unknowingly create.

Mindfulness and Presence as the Gateway to Liberation

The path to freedom, then, is one of mindfulness and presence. It is about realizing that thoughts are not permanent fixtures in our consciousness, but fleeting energy forms that can be observed and released. The more we practice being present—observing our thoughts without attachment or judgment—the more we begin to recognize that we are the awareness behind the thought. This awareness is liberating. As we detach from the ego and its endless stream of thoughts, we enter a state of pure consciousness where we are free from the limiting beliefs that once held us back.

The wisdom of spiritual leaders and prophets throughout history has echoed this truth. *Buddha*, for example, taught that the root of all suffering is attachment—attachment to our thoughts, our desires, and our identities. By letting go of these attachments, we can transcend the ego and experience true peace.

Jesus Christ spoke of the importance of forgiveness and self-awareness, encouraging us to look beyond the judgments of the mind and embrace love as the highest truth.

These teachings remind us that the ego's hold on our perception of reality is what keeps us in the cycle of suffering. Freedom, they say, comes when we release the grip of identification with the mind and return to the present moment, where true peace resides.

Living in Harmony with the Flow of Life

Ultimately, the lens through which we see the world is shaped by our thoughts. These thoughts are not inherently good or bad; rather, they are energy forms that we give power to through our identification with them.

By practicing mindfulness and detachment from the ego, we begin to see the world not as a reflection of our fears, but as a manifestation of the infinite possibilities that exist in the present moment. When we awaken to this truth, we step into our true power as conscious creators of our reality. The path to freedom is a practice of observing thoughts, understanding their fleeting nature, and realizing that we are not defined by them. By shifting our perception and returning to the present moment, we break free from the limitations of the ego and begin to live in harmony with the greater flow of life.

The world is not as it seems; it is as we perceive it. And when we change the way we see the world, we change the world itself.

Practice: The Power of Conscious Perception

In our everyday lives, we are constantly influenced by our thoughts, emotions, and external circumstances, which shape how we perceive the world. However, this perception is not a direct reflection of reality—it is filtered through the lens of our mind.

True freedom comes when we understand that our thoughts are not who we are, and we shift our perception to align with a higher state of awareness. By practicing mindfulness, detaching from the ego, and transforming negative thought patterns, we can reclaim our peace and experience life as a canvas of infinite possibilities.

The following practices will guide you in awakening to your true power as a conscious creator of your reality, helping you move beyond limiting beliefs and embrace a more expansive and empowering view of life.

Mindful Observation

This practice helps you step back and observe your thoughts without becoming attached to them. As you create space between yourself and your thoughts, you begin to recognize that you are the awareness behind them—not the thoughts themselves. This shift allows you to reclaim your power and gain clarity in your perception.

Find a quiet space and sit comfortably with your eyes closed. Focus on your breath to anchor yourself in the present moment. Allow thoughts to arise and pass by, as if they were clouds drifting through the sky. When a thought grabs your attention, gently bring your focus back to your breath, observing without judgment. Start with five minutes of this practice and gradually increase the time as you become more comfortable.

Detachment from Ego

Ego-driven thoughts often cloud our perception and trap us in limiting beliefs. The practice of detachment allows us to step outside of our thoughts and recognize that we are not defined by them. By disengaging from the ego's narrative, we free ourselves to experience reality as it truly is, rather than through the distortions of the mind. Throughout your day, pause when you notice a thought or emotion that feels defining (e.g., *I'm not good enough* or *I'm a failure)*. Ask yourself: *Who am I without this thought?* Notice how the attachment to the thought shifts or fades away as you detach from it. Remind yourself that you are the awareness behind your experiences, not the thoughts or emotions themselves.

Reframing Negative Thoughts

Negative thoughts shape our perception of reality. This practice empowers you to reframe limiting thoughts into more positive, empowering beliefs. By changing your mental framework, you begin to perceive opportunities instead of obstacles, shifting your view of the world and your role within it. When a negative thought arises (e.g., *I can't do this* or *This will never work)*, pause and replace it with a positive affirmation (e.g., *I am capable of overcoming challenges,* or *I am open to new possibilities)*. Reframe your thoughts multiple times a day, especially in moments of doubt or fear. As you repeat this process, you will begin to rewire your brain to default to positive, empowering beliefs.

Cultivating Gratitude

Gratitude shifts our focus from what's missing or wrong to what's abundant and good. By cultivating a mindset of gratitude, you raise your vibration and begin to see the world through a lens of abundance, which profoundly alters your perception of reality. Begin or end your day by writing down three things you are grateful for. As you reflect on each item, feel the positive emotions associated with it—appreciation, love, or joy. Over time, this practice will train your mind to focus on the positive aspects of life, shifting your perception to one of abundance.

The Present Moment

Presence is the doorway to freedom. The mind often wanders to the past or future, distorting our experience of the present moment. Practicing presence allows you to fully immerse yourself in the here and now, experiencing life as it truly is, without the overlay of past regrets or future anxieties. Engage in a simple activity, such as drinking water, walking, or washing dishes, and bring all of your attention to the task. Pay attention to the sensations, sights, and sounds around you without judgment or distraction. Whenever your mind drifts to the past or future, gently return your focus to the present moment. Practice presence in small moments throughout your day to strengthen your connection to the now.

The path to freedom lies in transforming how we perceive the world. Through mindfulness and detachment, we can break free from the limitations imposed by the ego and negative thought patterns.

As you engage in these practices, you will begin to notice a shift in your perception—less attachment to the mind's judgments and a greater awareness of your true nature. Over time, these practices will help you step into a higher state of consciousness, where the constraints of the ego dissolve, and the infinite possibilities of the present moment unfold.

As you change how you perceive yourself and the world, you begin to create a life of greater peace, freedom, and empowerment.

"Until you make the unconscious conscious, it will direct your life, and you will call it fate."[28]

—Carl Jung

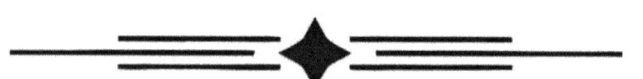

CHAPTER 18

EXPLORING AUTOHYPNOSIS: UNLOCKING THE POWER OF SELF-TRANSFORMATION

A*utohypnosis* is a powerful self-improvement technique that enables individuals to tap into the vast potential of their subconscious mind. Through focused attention, relaxation, and mental discipline, autohypnosis allows a person to enter a deeply relaxed and heightened state of awareness, which can then be harnessed for personal growth, healing, and change.

Unlike traditional hypnosis, which typically requires an external hypnotist or therapist, *autohypnosis* is self-induced, providing individuals with the freedom to engage in the process whenever and wherever they need it. This practice is rooted in the idea that the mind operates on both a conscious and subconscious level. While the conscious mind deals with everyday tasks and decisions, the subconscious mind governs automatic functions, habits, and deep-seated beliefs. By entering a focused state, *autohypnosis* bypasses the conscious mind and allows access to the subconscious, making it possible to introduce positive suggestions and make lasting changes. Whether used for reducing stress, overcoming negative habits, or improving mental clarity, *autohypnosis* offers a tool that is both empowering and transformative.

The Benefits of Autohypnosis

One of the most notable benefits is the ability to reduce stress and promote relaxation. In our fast-paced world, constant exposure to stressors can lead to a variety of physical and mental health issues, from anxiety to chronic pain. It offers a simple, effective method for counteracting these effects.

By inducing a state of deep relaxation, this practice lowers cortisol levels, calms the nervous system, and provides relief from stress. The ability to access this state of calm at will means that individuals can manage their stress levels proactively, rather than reacting to them after they've already escalated.

Another area where this practice proves invaluable is in overcoming negative habits and patterns. Many individuals embrace it as a means to break free from unhealthy behaviors, such as smoking, overeating, or procrastination. The process allows people to access their subconscious, where habits are deeply ingrained, and replace detrimental behaviors with positive ones. By repeating affirmations or visualizing healthier alternatives during a relaxed, focused state, individuals can reshape their responses and create new, supportive patterns of behavior.

Pain management is another area where *autohypnosis* has demonstrated its effectiveness. Chronic pain can be debilitating, both physically and emotionally, but this practice provides a way to manage and reduce the perception of pain.

Through focused attention and suggestion, *autohypnosis* can alter the brain's response to pain signals, offering relief and improving quality of life. Many people with conditions such as migraines, arthritis, or fibromyalgia find that regular practice helps them to manage their pain without relying on medication.

In addition to its physical benefits, it also enhances mental and emotional well-being. By improving one's ability to focus and concentrate, it can lead to increased productivity, creativity, and mental clarity. Whether preparing for a big presentation, tackling a challenging project, or simply needing a mental reset, *autohypnosis* can be used to sharpen focus and clear mental fog. For those struggling with anxiety or negative thought patterns, the ability to reprogram the subconscious mind can foster a sense of calm and self-confidence.

How Autohypnosis Works: The Science Behind It

"Every thought we think is creating our future."[29]*– Louise Hay*

The science behind *autohypnosis* is rooted in the understanding of how the brain processes relaxation, focus, and suggestion. When in a hypnotic state, brain activity shifts from the usual alert mode to a more relaxed and receptive state.

Studies have shown that hypnosis activates certain brain regions responsible for pain perception, emotional regulation, and relaxation. This shift in brain activity allows individuals to access deeper parts of the mind, facilitating change and personal growth. This practice works by shifting attention inward, away from the distractions of the external world, and focusing it on internal processes. This form of focused attention is a key aspect of hypnosis, whether it's guided by an external hypnotist or self-induced.

In a hypnotic state, the conscious mind takes a backseat, while the subconscious becomes more open to suggestions. This makes it easier to introduce new ideas, beliefs, and behaviors that align with personal goals, such as overcoming fears, building confidence, or healing from past trauma.

One of the most significant advantages is that it's a highly accessible tool. Unlike other therapeutic methods that require professional assistance, autohypnosis can be learned and practiced independently. Once an individual learns the basic techniques, they can incorporate autohypnosis into their daily routine as a self-help tool. This ability to control one's mental and emotional state without relying on external resources is a key factor in the widespread appeal of this practice.

Linking the *"I Am"* Meditation with Autohypnosis

"No man is free who is not master of himself."[30] – *Epictetus*

While *autohypnosis* offers a wealth of benefits, it's important to recognize that, like any practice, its effectiveness varies from person to person. Some individuals may find it more challenging to enter a deep state of relaxation or to maintain focus. However, with practice and patience, many people can master the technique and experience significant improvements in their lives. This is not a quick fix, but rather a skill that, when developed over time, can lead to lasting change.

The *"I Am"* meditation is a powerful mindfulness practice that centers around the affirmation of one's true essence or identity. By repeating the phrase *"I Am,"* practitioners focus on the present moment and align their thoughts with self-awareness, inner peace, and positive self-belief.

The essence of this meditation is to affirm and embrace one's inherent worth and purpose, fostering a deeper connection to the present and a sense of empowerment. This practice often involves repeating *"I Am"* followed by qualities, such as *I am calm, I am strong, or I am confident,* depending on the focus of the meditation. By using these affirmations, you reinforce a positive self-image and invite transformational change.

The *"I Am"* meditation can be seamlessly integrated into *autohypnosis* as both practices involve focused intention and deep relaxation to shift thought patterns and emotions. In *autohypnosis*, the goal is to bypass the critical conscious mind and directly influence the subconscious. By combining the *"I Am"* meditation's affirmations with autohypnosis, you enhance the impact of the affirmations, making them more potent as you enter a relaxed state where your subconscious is more receptive to positive suggestions.

In a world that often feels overwhelming and chaotic, autohypnosis provides a means of reclaiming control. It offers an opportunity to disconnect from external distractions and focus on what truly matters. Whether used to reduce stress, break harmful habits, manage pain, or improve mental clarity, *autohypnosis* is a versatile tool that can empower individuals to shape their own destinies.

By learning to tap into the subconscious mind, individuals can transform their lives from the inside out, gaining greater control over their thoughts, emotions, and actions.

Practice: Harnessing the Power of Autohypnosis

Autohypnosis is a powerful tool that allows individuals to access the subconscious mind and harness its vast potential for healing, growth, and transformation. By entering a deeply relaxed state, the conscious mind takes a back seat, allowing positive suggestions to reach the subconscious and create lasting change.

Here are some effective ways to incorporate *autohypnosis* into your daily life to help reduce stress, break negative habits, and enhance overall well-being.

Relaxation and Stress Relief

Begin by sitting or lying down in a quiet, comfortable space where you won't be disturbed. Close your eyes and take a few deep breaths, focusing on the feeling of air entering and leaving your body. This will help calm your mind and relax your body. Slowly scan your body, starting from your toes and working upward toward your head. With each area you mentally focus on, allow that part of your body to release any tension and relax fully. Once you feel deeply relaxed, repeat the affirmation: *I am calm and at peace with myself.* As you do, imagine a warm, soothing light filling your body, healing, and relaxing each muscle, leaving you completely at ease.

Breaking Negative Habits

Identify the specific habit you want to change, such as smoking, overeating, or procrastination. Acknowledge the impact this behavior has on your life and well-being. While in a relaxed state, visualize the habit in a neutral or negative light. See the consequences it has on your health, relationships, or life, and allow yourself to experience the discomfort associated with this behavior. Replace the negative behavior with a healthier alternative. Picture yourself making the positive choice, whether it's eating healthier, being more active, or staying focused on your work. See yourself empowered and in control, confidently making choices that align with your goals. Affirm to yourself: *I am in control of my actions and make choices that support my well-being.* Visualize living your new, healthier reality with ease and confidence.

Pain Management

Focus on the area of your body where you are experiencing pain. Allow your body to relax even further as you concentrate on this area, accepting the sensation without judgment. Visualize the pain as a color or shape. Imagine this representation of pain shrinking, transforming into a soothing sensation. Picture the discomfort dissolving and being replaced with a feeling of warmth and relief. Repeat the affirmation: *I am in control of my body and choose comfort and ease.* Picture the pain fading away completely, leaving you feeling calm, comfortable, and relaxed.

Enhancing Focus and Mental Clarity

Sit quietly in a comfortable position, take several deep breaths, and allow yourself to relax. Clear your mind of distractions and focus on your body's sensations. Visualize a task or goal you want to achieve. Picture yourself completing it with complete focus, feeling confident and clear. Imagine yourself working with ease, without any distractions, and seeing the task through to successful completion. As you continue to visualize, repeat the affirmation: *I am focused, clear, and capable of achieving my goals.* Visualize yourself succeeding, feeling proud of your accomplishments, and fully engaged in the task at hand.

Building Confidence and Self-Empowerment

While in a relaxed state, recall a time in your life when you felt proud and confident. It could be a specific achievement, a moment of success, or any time you felt truly capable and strong.

Relive this moment in your mind, focusing on the positive emotions and feelings of strength that you experienced. Feel those empowering emotions as if they are happening in the present moment. Repeat the affirmation: *I am confident, capable, and worthy of success.* Visualize yourself succeeding in future situations, feeling empowered, resilient, and capable of overcoming any challenge with grace.

Autohypnosis is a versatile and effective technique that can help individuals transform their lives from the inside out. By integrating the *"I Am"* meditation you can amplify the power of positive affirmations and tap into the deep potential of your subconscious mind. This combination fosters lasting transformation by reprogramming limiting beliefs and empowering you to create the life you desire with confidence and clarity.

Through regular practice, you can develop a deeper connection to your true self and unlock your full potential.

"The records don't dictate what to do but empower us with insights to create positive change. They help release self-limiting beliefs, transform relationships, and foster inner and outer harmon"[31]

—*Bhavya Gaur*

CHAPTER 19

AKASHIC RECORDS: A GATEWAY TO INFINITE KNOWLEDGE

The *Akashic Records*, often called the *"Book of Life,"* is an esoteric concept describing a metaphysical repository of knowledge containing all the details of each soul's journey. Spiritual teacher *Bhavya Gaur* describes the *Akashic Records* as a source of compassionate guidance, offering clarity to help individuals heal, grow, and embrace a life of peace.

The Records are thought to hold every thought, emotion, intention, action, and event of each soul, recorded as vibrational frequencies within a non-physical dimension. It is often described as a vast, energetic database in which every individual has their own unique *"soul book,"* chronicling their past lives, present experiences, and even future potential.

Based on my personal experience of connecting with *The Records* over the past ten years, this metaphysical archive is seen not merely as a storage of information but as a powerful guidance tool that can influence our perceptions, emotions, and understanding of reality.

Edgar Cayce, who was considered a pioneer of the modern *New Age* movement, described the *Akashic Records* as " *God's book of remembrance.*" He explained: " *Upon time and space is written the thoughts, the deeds, the activities of an entity—as in relationships to its environs, its hereditary influence; as directed – or judgment drawn by or according to what the entity's ideal is.* "[32]

Some spiritual perspectives suggest that the *Akashic Records* are composed of a universal energy called *"Akasha,"* a Sanskrit term meaning *"hidden"* or *"secret space,"* with roots in the word *"kāś,"* which translates to *"to be."* This energy is believed to encompass all that exists, spanning time and space, and is stored on a metaphysical plane known as the ethereal realm. Many believe that accessing the *Akashic Records* is possible for anyone, though some schools of thought argue it requires specific training. Regardless, practitioners generally agree that these records are neutral and objective, simply recording what has occurred and what is, without assigning moral judgments or distinctions of right and wrong.

Understanding the Akashic Records—A Journey Beyond Time and Space

In our 3D human experience, we're conditioned to think in linear terms of past, present, and future. However, the *Akashic Records* transcend these limitations, existing beyond time and space. They are believed to be in a dimension where all moments—past, present, and potential futures—exist simultaneously, offering a more fluid perspective on time and growth.

Each soul's journey is recorded and preserved in these realms, allowing individuals to access profound knowledge, insight, and healing. Through the *Records,* we can explore the karmic lessons of past lifetimes, understand current life patterns, and open ourselves to growth and expansion in alignment with our highest self.

By tapping into the *Akashic Records,* people seek to understand their soul's purpose, resolve life challenges, and release energies or experiences that no longer serve them. This exploration can help us align more closely with our true path, empowering us to experience life with greater clarity, peace, and purpose.

The Theosophical Connection

In the late 19th century, *Helena Blavatsky* became a prominent figure in a new spiritual philosophy called Theosophy. Drawing on Western esoteric traditions and Eastern philosophies, Theosophy proposed that an ancient brotherhood of enlightened Masters held the wisdom of humanity's spiritual evolution. *Blavatsky* introduced the concept of the *Akashic Records*, which she described as *"tablets of astral light."*[33] *Alfred Percy Sinnett*, a contemporary of *Blavatsky* and fellow Theosophist, later coined the term *"Akashic Records."*[34]

By the early 20th century, Austrian philosopher *Rudolf Steiner*, also a Theosophist, expanded on the concept, claiming to access the *Akashic Records* through his clairvoyant abilities. *Steiner* said this knowledge provided insights into cosmic truths, including events from *Jesus Christ's* life not recorded in scripture, which he referred to as the *"Fifth Gospel."*[35]

Accessing the Akashic Records

Accessing the *Akashic Records* is believed to be an intuitive or spiritual process, often involving meditative techniques or visualization. While some people consult trained *Akashic Records* practitioners, anyone can learn to enter this realm by cultivating a practice rooted in reverence, trust, and openness. To access the *Records*, many practitioners use a prayer or mantra to attune themselves to its vibrational frequency.

Quieting the mind, entering a state of deep meditation, and setting an intention are important steps. The experience is often described as receiving impressions, feelings, and insights rather than specific words or images. These insights are usually subtle and can feel like an internal knowing or a gentle nudge guiding you toward clarity.

One of the most powerful aspects is their role in our soul's evolution. Through understanding past experiences and recognizing repeated patterns, we can address and release karmic imprints that may be holding us back.

This allows us to elevate our consciousness and engage in more fulfilling and purposeful ways. It's an opportunity to integrate life lessons, evolve spiritually, and consciously choose a path of growth and enlightenment.

The *Records* encourage us to see our lives from a higher perspective, where each experience—joyful or challenging—serves as a stepping stone for greater spiritual development. Our individual *"soul books"* are filled with stories that teach resilience, compassion, and unconditional love. As we read these chapters, we understand that each situation is divinely orchestrated to help us remember our innate potential, moving us closer to the realization of our full essence.

Practice: Unlocking the Wisdom of Your Akashic Records

Accessing the *Akashic Records* can provide deep insights into your life purpose, relationships, and spiritual growth.

If you feel drawn to explore this spiritual resource, these simple practices can help you connect with the *Akashic* field, opening a doorway to profound self-awareness and transformation.

Meditative Visualization to Access Your Soul's Book

Find a quiet place where you can sit comfortably and remain undisturbed. Close your eyes, take a few deep breaths, and allow yourself to relax, releasing any tension in your body.

Setting Your Intention

Silently or aloud, state your intention to connect with your soul's journey through the *Akashic Records*. You might say: *I am open to receiving insight and guidance from my Akashic Records, in alignment with my highest good and soul evolution.*

Visualization

Imagine yourself standing before a grand, ancient library filled with glowing books. Each book represents a soul, and the energy of peace and wisdom fills the space. Visualize yourself walking through this library until you come across a special book that feels like it's meant for you—this is your soul's book. Imagine this book glowing warmly, waiting for you to open it.

Opening the Book

When you feel ready, reach out and open the book. Take note of any sensations, emotions, or thoughts that arise. Sometimes you might see colors, feel emotions, or even hear words—trust whatever arises, as each impression is meaningful.

Begin to ask gentle questions, such as:

What is a lesson my soul is learning in this lifetime?

Are there any patterns I'm ready to release?

What qualities should I embrace for my soul's growth?

Receiving and Integrating

Take time to receive any answers or impressions without judgment. Write down any insights, messages, or feelings that come to you, knowing that even subtle impressions can have profound meaning. Express gratitude for the experience and the wisdom shared with you and imagine yourself closing your soul's book with a sense of peace and gratitude.

Returning

Visualize yourself gently leaving the library and returning to your physical space, bringing with you the sense of peace and clarity gained from the experience.

Grounding Afterward

Ensure you return to the physical world fully present and balanced. Close the session by thanking the *Akashic Records* and any spiritual guides you encountered. Visualize yourself disconnecting from the energy of the records and returning to the here and now. Perform grounding exercises, such as walking barefoot on the earth or holding a grounding crystal-like hematite or black tourmaline.

Repeated Practice for Mastery

Dedicate regular time to explore the *Akashic Records*. Weekly sessions can help you refine your ability to access and interpret the guidance received. Experiment with different methods, such as guided meditations, working with a teacher, or incorporating intuitive tools like tarot or oracle cards for added insight.

Integrating Guidance into Daily Life

Reflect on the guidance received and identify specific steps you can take to implement it. For example, if the *Records* suggest letting go of a limiting belief, focus on affirmations or seek supportive practices like therapy or mindfulness to release it. Keep track of changes and growth in your journal to recognize the impact of working with the Akashic Records.

Exploring Past Lives

Set a specific intention, such as: *I wish to understand a past life experience that influences my current relationships.* Visualize stepping into a timeline or storybook and allowing details of a past life to unfold. Pay attention to emotions, settings, and recurring themes.

Working with Spirit Guides

During meditation, invite a spirit guide, angel, or ascended master to assist in interpreting the *Akashic Records.* Ask specific questions and remain open to their symbolic or energetic responses.

Cultivating a Heart-Centered Approach

Begin each session by focusing on your heart chakra, visualizing it glowing with light. Remember that the guidance received is rooted in unconditional love, offering insights to empower and uplift you.

These practices can help you feel connected to your soul's journey, receive guidance, and engage with your own wisdom. Through the *Akashic Records,* we are reminded that we are far more than our human experiences. We are timeless, connected beings with endless potential for growth, learning, and transformation.

"Just for today, I will not be angry. Just for today, I will not worry. Just for today, I will do my work honestly. Just for today, I will be grateful. Just for today, I will be kind to every living thing. "[36]

—Dr. Mikao Usui (founder of Reiki)

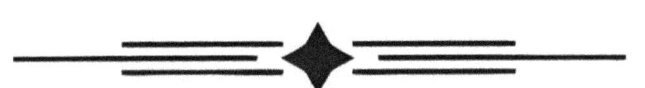

CHAPTER 20

THE BENEFITS AND MEANING OF REIKI: BRIDGING SKEPTICISM AND UNDERSTANDING

R*eiki,* originating from Japan, is an ancient form of energy healing that involves the transfer of universal life force energy through the practitioner's hands to the recipient. The word *"Reiki"* combines two Japanese words: *Rei,* meaning *"universal"* or *"spiritual,"* and *Ki,* meaning *"life force energy"* or *"vital energy."*

This practice aims to balance the body's energy centers, promote relaxation, and facilitate self-healing. In Eastern cultures, the concept of energy flow is integral to understanding health and well-being. Practices like acupuncture, herbal medicine, and Tai Chi are based on maintaining and restoring this flow. In the West, however, the idea of *"energy"* in health is less familiar, contributing to skepticism surrounding *Reiki.* Western medical paradigms emphasize physical, measurable phenomena, often overlooking subtle energy systems. Therefore, *Reiki*'s intangible nature makes it challenging to accept. However, its core principles resonate with natural, instinctive healing processes we all engage in—processes I've personally deepened through over twenty years of practice as a certified *Reiki Master.*

Hands-On Healing—An Innate Response

Think about what we naturally do when we experience physical pain, such as twisting an ankle or bumping a knee. Instinctively, we place our hands on the affected area. This simple act serves multiple purposes. Placing hands on the injured area helps us focus our mental energy directly on the site of trauma. This concentrated awareness facilitates a stronger mind-body connection, promoting healing.

The hands' gentle warmth and contact can also help soothe the nervous system, reducing stress and inflammation—factors that hinder recovery. This unconscious act of self-soothing is essentially a form of *Reiki.* By channeling attention and calm energy to the site of pain, we create an optimal environment for the body's natural healing mechanisms to function effectively.

This practice offers a range of benefits. It promotes relaxation and reduces stress by activating the parasympathetic nervous system, fostering a calm, restful state. Healing occurs most effectively when the body is relaxed, much like during deep sleep, when the conscious mind and its distractions get out of the way. It also supports physical healing by enhancing blood flow, reducing inflammation, and accelerating tissue repair. The focused awareness and calm state induced by *Reiki* enable the body to direct resources efficiently to the area of need.

Beyond physical health, this practice addresses emotional and psychological well-being as emotional traumas and stress often manifest as energy blockages in the body. By releasing these blockages, *Reiki* can offer relief from anxiety, depression, and emotional distress.

Practitioners provide a neutral, supportive space, helping clients confront and process emotional pain safely. Additionally, *Reiki* enhances the mind-body connection by encouraging mindfulness. Recipients often gain insights into their emotional or physical state, fostering greater self-awareness and overall well-being.

Addressing Skepticism with Practical Explanations

Skeptics may dismiss *Reiki* as pseudoscience, but its principles align with fundamental concepts of psychology, physiology, and neuroscience. The power of focused attention in healing is well-recognized in psychological practices.

Mindfulness, a widely accepted technique, operates on a similar principle—directing awareness inward to promote well-being. The placebo effect, often cited dismissively, demonstrates the mind's profound ability to influence physical health. Its calming presence and focused attention may harness this effect, encouraging the body to heal itself.

One significant barrier for skeptics is the association of *Reiki* with crystals, rituals, and spiritual beliefs. While these tools can enhance a practice, they are not essential. At its core, this practice is about simple, human connection and energy transfer. By presenting this practice in a neutral, non-dogmatic way, we make it accessible to a broader audience, emphasizing its practical benefits over esoteric symbolism. This approach helps cast a wider net, inviting more people to experience the healing potential of *Reiki* without feeling alienated by unfamiliar practices.

Rediscovering an Ancient Wisdom

There are three level of *Reiki* training: *Level 1 - Shoden (The First Teachings), Level 2- Okuden (The Inner Teachings)* and *Level 3- Shinpiden (Master Level or Mystery Teachings).* One of the most beautiful aspects is its inclusivity. Anyone can learn and practice *Reiki,* regardless of their age, background, or belief system. There's no need for special abilities or prior experience with energy work. The atonement process simply reconnects individuals with the universal energy that flows through all living beings.

Reiki operates on the principle that we are all naturally connected to this life force energy. The training process helps individuals become aware of this connection and use it intentionally for healing and well-being. Unlike some other spiritual or healing practices, this practice doesn't require elaborate rituals or specific tools.

The primary *"instrument"* is the practitioner's intention, hands, and presence. While the *Master Level* represents the highest formal training, true mastery is an ongoing journey of personal growth and self-discovery. Practicing *Reiki* regularly deepens one's connection to the energy and enhances intuitive abilities. Many *Reiki Masters* continue to learn and integrate other healing modalities, strengthening their practice and expanding their understanding. Throughout my personal journey, I have explored Angelic healing, Akashic Records reading, EFT practice, autohypnosis, yoga and meditation, integrating these practices as additional tools.

In essence, this practice is a lifelong journey. Each session—whether practicing *self-Reiki* or working with others—offers new insights and healing opportunities. The simplicity and accessibility of *Reiki* make it a powerful tool for personal transformation, fostering well-being, inner peace, and a deeper connection to life.

Reiki is not a foreign, mystical practice—it's a natural, intuitive form of healing we've always known. By fostering relaxation, focus, and a strong mind-body connection, it offers a powerful tool for self-healing and well-being. To skeptics, the invitation is simple: approach with an open mind and experience it firsthand.

Its benefits, while intangible, are deeply felt and universally accessible. In a world of constant stress and disconnection, this practice serves as a reminder of our inherent capacity to heal and reconnect with ourselves.

Practice: Cultivating Inner Healing and Balance Through Reiki

Reiki offers a profound yet simple approach to healing and self-care, deeply rooted in natural human instincts. Practicing *Reiki* doesn't require special tools or elaborate rituals; it's about reconnecting with the universal energy and fostering mindfulness.

Here are some practical exercises that embody these principles, encouraging a deeper connection with oneself and the healing process.

Self-Reiki for Daily Healing

Self-Reiki is an excellent starting point for anyone, regardless of their experience level. It allows you to connect with your own energy, calm the mind, and promote well-being.

Preparation: Sit or lie down in a comfortable position. Take a few deep breaths to center yourself.

Hand Placement: Gently place your hands on or near different parts of your body, starting with the crown of your head. Move to your forehead, throat, chest, stomach, and then legs. Hold each position for a few minutes.

Focus and Awareness: As you rest your hands on each area, bring your awareness to the sensations. Notice warmth, tingling, or any energy flow. If your mind wanders, gently bring your focus back to your breath and the area you're treating.

Completion: After you've covered the whole body, place your hands on your heart and take a few moments to express gratitude for the session. This exercise mirrors the innate healing response, where placing hands on an injured area draws attention and facilitates recovery.

Healing Hands for Others

You don't need to be a certified *Reiki* practitioner to share energy with others. A simple act of presence and intention can be powerful.

Ask for Permission: Always ensure the person is open to receiving energy work.

Comfortable Position: Have the person sit or lie down in a relaxed environment.

Hand Positioning: Gently place your hands on key areas like the shoulders, head, or back or simply hover them slightly above the body. Focus on maintaining a calm and neutral presence.

Maintain Neutrality: As mentioned, a non-judgmental, supportive mindset creates a safe space. Avoid projecting thoughts or expectations onto the recipient. Simply "hold space" for them. This practice exemplifies the power of human connection and focused attention in healing, resonating with the

core principles of *Reiki* and addressing the skepticism about its efficacy.

Mindfulness Meditation with Reiki

Combining mindfulness and *Reiki* enhances self-awareness and relaxation.

Sit Comfortably: Close your eyes and focus on your breath.

Hand Placement: Rest your hands on your lap or over your heart.

Visualize Energy: With each inhale, visualize a gentle light filling your body. With each exhale, imagine releasing tension or negative energy.

Silent Affirmation: Repeat affirmations like: *I am open to healing, or I allow energy to flow freely through me.* This practice aligns with the mind-body connection central to Reiki, where focused awareness promotes physical and emotional healing.

Reiki for Emotional Healing

Reiki can help address emotional blockages or distress.

Identify the Emotion: Reflect on the emotional pain or trauma you want to release.

Heart-Centered Healing: Place your hands over your heart or stomach. Close your eyes and breathe deeply.

Observe and Release: Allow any emotions to surface without judgment. Imagine the energy of those emotions dissolving or being released with each breath.

Hold Space for Yourself: Treat yourself with kindness and compassion, embodying the neutral, supportive space that *Reiki* offers. This mirrors the emotional processing described earlier, where practitioners help clients confront and release deep-seated issues safely.

At Level 3, a *Reiki Master* gains access to all *Reiki* symbols, including the powerful Master symbol. These symbols are sacred tools that amplify energy, facilitate focus, and serve as keys to different aspects of healing. True mastery in *Reiki* extends beyond technical skills; it involves living by *Reiki*'s principles, such as compassion, gratitude, and mindfulness. A *Reiki Master* serves as both a healer and a guide, continuously deepening their understanding while helping others discover their healing potential.

By practicing and teaching from a place of openness and authenticity, *Reiki Masters* bridge the gap between ancient wisdom and modern life, demonstrating that its profound benefits are accessible to all who seek healing and connection.

These practical exercises demonstrate that *Reiki* is not an abstract or esoteric concept but a natural part of human experience.

Approaching it with openness and neutrality, as discussed, allows people to rediscover their innate capacity to heal, fostering a deeper connection with themselves and the universal energy that surrounds

"The greatest gift you can give yourself is the gift of understanding your emotions. "[37]
—*Thich Nhat Hanh*

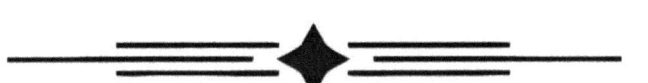

CHAPTER 21

EMOTIONAL FREEDOM TECHNIQUE (EFT): UNLOCKING EMOTIONAL HEALING THROUGH TAPPING

E*motional Freedom Technique (EFT)*, widely known as tapping, has emerged as a powerful approach for addressing emotional distress, reducing stress, and promoting healing. Rooted in the principles of ancient Chinese medicine and modern psychology, this practice bridges the gap between mind and body, offering a holistic approach to well-being. This simple yet profound practice is gaining recognition not only for its effectiveness in alleviating emotional pain but also for its accessibility and ease of integration into everyday life.

EFT operates on the premise that unresolved emotional issues disrupt the body's energy system, leading to both emotional and physical symptoms. This concept stems from traditional Chinese medicine, which views health as the result of balanced energy (qi or chi) flowing through meridian channels. When this energy becomes blocked or imbalanced, it can manifest as anxiety, stress, chronic pain, or emotional turmoil.

In the context of modern neuroscience, its effectiveness can be linked to its impact on the brain's amygdala—the region responsible for the fight-or-flight response. When we experience stress or trauma, the amygdala triggers this response, flooding the body with stress hormones like cortisol.

While this mechanism is essential for survival, chronic activation can lead to anxiety, emotional reactivity, and even physical illness. Tapping helps deactivate this response, sending a calming signal to the brain and reducing stress.

Emotional Healing: Beyond Talk Therapy

Traditional talk therapy has long been a cornerstone of mental health care, offering a safe space to process emotions and gain insight. However, many individuals find that simply discussing their issues doesn't always lead to lasting change. *EFT* addresses this gap by incorporating the body into the healing process.

By focusing on the physical sensations associated with emotions and gently tapping on specific points, individuals engage both their minds and bodies, creating a more comprehensive healing experience. This embodied approach helps break the cycle of chronic stress and negative thinking patterns. Many people report feeling an immediate sense of relief and relaxation after tapping, even when dealing with long-standing issues. This is particularly significant for those who feel *"stuck"* in their healing journey, as this practice provides a tangible method to release trapped emotions and move forward.

One of the most compelling aspects of this practice is its versatility. It can be used to address a wide range of issues, including anxiety, depression, phobias, chronic pain, and even performance anxiety. For example, frontline workers during the COVID-19 pandemic found it helpful in managing the immense stress and emotional burden of their roles. By incorporating tapping into their routines before and after shifts, they were able to ground themselves, release tension, and maintain emotional resilience.

EFT's benefits extend beyond emotional well-being to physical health. Emotional stress often manifests as physical symptoms—headaches, back pain, digestive issues, and fatigue. By addressing the underlying emotional causes, tapping can alleviate these physical manifestations, promoting overall wellness. It also fosters greater emotional awareness and self-regulation. Through the process of identifying specific issues and acknowledging their emotional impact, individuals develop a deeper understanding of their emotional landscape. This increased self-awareness enables more conscious responses to life's challenges, reducing reactivity and fostering a sense of inner calm.

The Simplicity and Accessibility of EFT

One of *EFT*'s greatest strengths is, similar with *Reiki,* its accessibility. Unlike some therapeutic interventions that require specialized knowledge or resources, tapping can be practiced by anyone, anywhere. It doesn't require elaborate tools or rituals—just an open mind and a willingness to engage with one's emotions. This simplicity makes it a powerful tool for self-care, allowing individuals to take an active role in their healing journey. Its non-invasive nature makes it suitable for people of all ages and backgrounds.

Whether dealing with minor daily stresses or deep-seated trauma, anyone can benefit from tapping. Its gentle, affirming approach encourages self-compassion, reminding individuals that it's safe to acknowledge and release difficult emotions.

A Holistic Path to Emotional Freedom

EFT represents a shift in how we approach emotional healing. By recognizing the interconnectedness of mind and body, it offers a more holistic and effective path to well-being. This approach aligns with the growing awareness in both Eastern and Western medicine that true healing involves addressing not just the mind but the entire being.

In a world where stress and emotional disconnection are prevalent, this practice serves as a reminder of our innate capacity to heal and reconnect with ourselves. It empowers individuals to break free from the patterns that hold them back, fostering resilience, self-awareness, and inner peace.

Ultimately, this practice is more than just a therapeutic tool—it's a journey of self-discovery and transformation. By engaging both mind and body, it offers a powerful pathway to emotional freedom, helping individuals tap into their full potential for healing and well-being.

Practice: Emotional Freedom Technique as a Path to Inner Healing

EFT or tapping, offers a gentle yet transformative approach to emotional and physical well-being. By combining mindful awareness with physical stimulation of meridian points, EFT helps release trapped emotions, reduce stress, and promote inner calm.

The following exercises provide a gateway to reconnect with your emotions and body, empowering you to face life's challenges with greater resilience and peace.

Releasing Stress and Anxiety

Identify the Emotion: Choose a specific stressor or anxious thought.

Intensity Rating: Rate the intensity on a scale of 0 to 10.

Affirmation: Tap the side of your hand while saying: *Even though I feel this stress, I deeply and completely accept myself.*

Tapping Sequence: Move through the standard tapping points:

Eyebrow (EB): *This stress I'm feeling...*

Side of Eye (SE): *I feel overwhelmed by...*

Under Eye (UE): *This anxiety in my body...*

Under Nose (UN): *I acknowledge these feelings...*

Chin (CH): *It's hard to let go of this stress...*

Collarbone (CB): *But I'm open to finding peace...*

Under Arm (UA): *Releasing the tension in my body...*

Top of Head (TH): *I choose to feel calm and safe.*

Repeat and Reassess: After one or two rounds, take a deep breath and reassess your intensity rating. Repeat until you feel significant relief.

Letting Go of Emotional Blocks

Identify the Block: Reflect on a recurring negative feeling or thought pattern.

Affirmation: Tap the side of your hand while saying: *Even though I feel stuck in this emotion, I choose to release it now.*

Tapping Points Affirmations:

Eyebrow: *I feel this emotional block...*

Side of Eye: *It has been with me for a long time...*

Under Eye: *I recognize this feeling and its hold on me...*

Under Nose: *I'm ready to let it go...*

Chin: *I am safe to release this now...*

Collarbone: *I choose to release this block and invite healing...*

Under Arm: *I am open to emotional freedom...*

Top of Head: *I welcome peace and clarity into my life.*

Pain and Physical Discomfort Relief

Identify the Pain: Focus on the specific area of discomfort.

Intensity Rating: Rate the pain level from 0 to 10.

Affirmation: Tap the side of your hand, saying: *Even though I have this pain, I deeply love and accept myself.*

Tapping Points Affirmations:

Eyebrow: *This pain in my [location]...*

Side of Eye: *It's affecting my peace...*

Under Eye: *I acknowledge this discomfort...*

Under Nose: *My body is holding this tension...*

Chin: *I choose to let it release...*

Collarbone: *Inviting comfort and healing to this area...*

Under Arm: *I feel the tension easing...*

Top of Head: *I allow my body to relax and heal.*

Reassess: After a few rounds, check in with your body to notice changes in pain intensity.

Cultivating Daily Calm and Resilience

Morning Grounding: Start the day by setting an intention with a quick tapping sequence: *I release yesterday's worries and* *embrace today's possibilities. I am grounded, centered, and ready for whatever comes my way.*

Evening Reflection: Before bed, clear the day's stress:

Releasing Fear and Building Confidence:

Identify a Fear: Name a specific fear or self-doubt.

Tapping Affirmations:

Eyebrow: *I feel afraid of...*

Side of Eye: *This fear has held me back...*

Under Eye: *But I choose to face it now...*

Under Nose: *I am stronger than this fear...*

Chin: *I release this fear from my body...*

Collarbone: *I invite courage and confidence...*

Top of Head: I choose to trust myself.

EFT is a powerful tool for releasing emotional blockages and reducing physical discomfort by tapping on specific meridian points. It helps rewire the subconscious mind, allowing for the release of negative emotions and limiting beliefs.

Regular practice promotes emotional resilience, mental clarity, and a deeper sense of well-being. By integrating tapping into your daily routine, you can foster a greater connection to yourself and handle life's challenges with calm and balance.

Over time, this practice empowers individuals to break free from emotional burdens and create lasting emotional freedom.

"*The more you meditate,*
the more helpful you can be to others.
Without meditation, you are not going beyond
the physical body."[38]
—*Swami Vivekananda*

CHAPTER 22

THE LIFE-CHANGING BENEFITS OF MEDITATION: A JOURNEY WITHIN

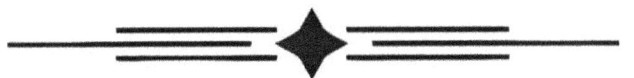

I truly believe if we understood the profoundly transformative power of meditation, we would never miss a single day of practice for the rest of our life. This ancient practice is much more than a tool for relaxation—it is a gateway to self-discovery, healing, and personal growth. Meditation connects us to our higher selves, fosters emotional resilience, enhances focus, and creates a deep sense of interconnectedness with the world.

Meditation's benefits extend far beyond stress reduction, empowering you to face life's challenges with grace and wisdom Once touched by the inner peace and clarity that meditation brings, you will never want to live without it. It reconnects you with your soul, aligns you with your higher self, and fosters a sense of unity with others and the universe.

Meditation offers a variety of practices that cater to different needs and preferences. From morning meditations that set intentions for the day to evening meditations focused on relaxation and gratitude, each practice brings its unique benefits. Other forms, such as mindfulness meditation, transcendental meditation, and loving-kindness meditation, help to cultivate presence, compassion, and emotional well-being.

Building a Sustainable Meditation Practice and Exploring Different Types of Meditation

Establishing a meditation routine requires patience and consistency. Start small, dedicating 5-10 minutes daily to sitting in stillness. As your body and mind adjust to the practice, gradually increase the duration. Choose a style that resonates with you—be it mindfulness, mantra-based meditation, or guided visualization—and explore what works best. Creating a sacred space for meditation can also enhance the experience. A quiet corner with calming elements like soft lighting, soothing scents, or inspirational decor can make meditation a cherished part of your day.

There are many styles of meditation, each with unique benefits and techniques. It can be valuable to explore various forms to find the practices that resonate most with you.

Mindfulness Meditation: This involves focusing on the present moment without judgment, often by observing the breath or doing a body scan. Mindfulness can be incorporated into daily life, helping you anchor in the present moment.

Loving-Kindness Meditation: This meditation nurtures compassion by encouraging positive thoughts toward yourself and others. By silently repeating phrases like *May I be happy, may I be peaceful* and extending these intentions to others, you cultivate a heart full of kindness.

Transcendental Meditation (TM): TM involves silently repeating a mantra to help access a state of deep relaxation and consciousness. Often practiced with eyes closed in a quiet space, this technique can be deeply calming.

Movement Meditation: Combining physical activity with mindfulness, movement meditation brings awareness to the body. This could be yoga, tai chi, qi gong, walking, or even mindful running—any activity that helps you stay present and connected with your body, combining movement with mindfulness at the same time.

Zen Meditation (Zazen): This is a seated meditation, typically practiced in stillness and silence, focusing on the breath and clearing the mind. It's a practice of simply *"being"* without attachment to thoughts or emotions.

Vipassana Meditation: A form of meditation that translates to *"insight"* or *"clear seeing,"* Vipassana is a silent, observation-based meditation. Rather than avoiding sensory input, it encourages practitioners to observe everything around them with complete presence and stillness.

Other types of meditations that can be explored: *sound healing meditation, chakra meditation, kundalini meditation, yoga nidra, tonglen meditation, body-scan meditation, guided visualization, self-inquiry (Atma Vichara), Christian Contemplative Prayer* etc.

Numerous studies confirm the remarkable benefits of meditation for physical, emotional, mental, and spiritual well-being. It enhances our sense of purpose, deepens self-awareness, and fosters personal transformation through improved clarity and focus. It has been shown to reduce depression, boost creativity, strengthen the immune system, improve sleep quality, and lower blood pressure.

The Profound Impact of Meditation

"The quieter you become, the more you can hear."[39]*- Ram Das*
Through meditation, we can reshape our thoughts and actions, cultivating a reality grounded in peace, balance, and love. Meditation is not merely a practice; it is a way of life—an ongoing journey of self-discovery, healing, and growth that

transforms every aspect of our existence. It is not about escaping reality but rather about awakening to it with clarity and compassion.

There are two primary approaches to meditation. The first involves retreating into stillness, shutting out the external world, and repeating mantras to quiet the mind. The second, found in practices like Vipassana and Zen, seeks to find peace amidst activity. These practices teach us to remain centered and calm while engaging with the world through all our senses.

Meditation is not a destination but a lifelong journey of growth and discovery. With each session, we unlock deeper levels of awareness and expand our capacity for love, wisdom, and peace. Its benefits ripple into every area of life, transforming our relationships, career, and health. It is a tool that empowers us to live more fully, authentically, and joyfully.

This practice holds the power to transform our lives from the inside out. Through self-discovery, healing, and mindfulness, it helps us navigate the complexities of life with grace and purpose. Whether you're just beginning your meditation journey or deepening an existing practice, the benefits are profound and far-reaching.

By embracing meditation as a daily practice, you invite lasting change, inner peace, and the boundless potential to live a life aligned with your highest self.

Practice: Self-Discovery, Healing and Growth through Meditation

Meditation has evolved into a diverse practice, offering various techniques that cater to different needs and preferences. Each type of meditation serves a unique purpose, whether it's calming the mind, fostering self-awareness, or cultivating compassion.

Below is an exploration of popular meditation types and what they offer, along with practical ideas on how to incorporate them into your life. To experience the powerful benefits of this practice, consistency is key. Start small, with a few minutes each day, and gradually increase your practice as it becomes a natural part of your routine.

The following is a simple guide to establishing a meditation practice that can fit into your daily life.

Morning Intention Meditation

Begin your day by setting a positive intention. With each breath, visualize your intention manifesting, such as peace, productivity, or compassion. As you breathe in, imagine drawing energy from the universe to fuel this intention. As you exhale, release any doubts, fears, or negativity. Silently affirm your intention: *Today, I am peaceful and present,* or whatever resonates with you.

Midday Mindfulness Practice

Use this practice to center yourself, especially during a busy day. Find a quiet spot or pause wherever you are. Focus on your breath, letting it anchor you in the present moment. As thoughts or emotions arise, observe them without judgment. Let them pass like clouds in the sky. This can be done with eyes open, observing surroundings, or closed for deeper focus.

Evening Gratitude Meditation

At the end of the day, find a quiet space to reflect on moments of gratitude. Bring to mind three things you are thankful for, no matter how small. Visualize these moments, allowing a sense of warmth and appreciation to fill you with each breath. Let your body and mind settle into a state of peace, releasing any tension or stress from the day.

Loving-Kindness Meditation

Once or twice a week, practice sending love and compassion to yourself and others. Start by repeating phrases for yourself, such as: *May I be happy, may I be safe, may I be free from suffering.*

Gradually extend these wishes to loved ones, acquaintances, and eventually to all beings. This meditation fosters compassion, kindness, and empathy, strngthening your bond with the world.

Mindfulness Meditation

Sit comfortably and focus on your breath.

Observe any sensations in your body or thoughts that arise, simply acknowledging them without judgment. Gently bring your focus back to the breath when your mind wanders. This can also be practiced throughout the day in daily activities, such as eating or walking.

Body-Scan Meditation

Lie down or sit in a relaxed position. Close your eyes and take a few deep breaths. Start at your toes and work your way up to your head, bringing awareness to each body part. Notice any areas of tension and consciously relax them with each breath.

Transcendental Meditation (TM)

Sit comfortably with your eyes closed. Repeat a chosen mantra silently in your mind. Continue repeating the mantra for 15-20 minutes, twice a day. The repetition of the mantra helps transcend ordinary thoughts and access a deeper state of consciousness.

Zen Meditation (Zazen)

Sit in a comfortable, upright position, either on a cushion (zafu) or a chair. Focus on your breath or simply observe the thoughts and sensations that arise. Let thoughts come and go without engaging or trying to control them. Practice for 20 minutes or longer to develop a sense of deep peace and clarity.

Vipassana Meditation

Sit in a comfortable position and focus on your breath.

As you breathe, observe the sensations in your body and the arising thoughts, emotions, and perceptions. Try not to judge or react to these experiences, just observe them with clarity.

Continue observing your body and mind for an extended period to deepen your awareness.

Movement Meditation

Engage in a movement practice such as yoga, tai chi, or mindful walking. Focus on the sensations of your body moving, paying attention to how your body feels in each posture or step.

Let go of all distractions and fully immerse yourself in the act of movement, using the rhythm of your body to stay present.

Guided Meditation (Varies)

Choose a guided meditation from an app, website, or recording.

Follow the instructions provided, allowing yourself to relax, focus, and engage with the visualization or specific prompts. Guided meditations can address specific goals, such as stress reduction, relaxation, or self-empowerment.

Sound Meditation

Sit in a comfortable position with your eyes closed. Listen to soothing sounds such as bells, gongs, or nature sounds, or use chanting or music. Focus on how the sound feels in your body, noticing the vibrations and resonance. Let the sound guide you into a deeper state of relaxation.

Visualization Meditation

Close your eyes and visualize a peaceful scene, such as a beach or forest, or focus on a personal goal. Imagine the colors, sounds, and smells in detail. Use your senses to fully immerse yourself in the visualization, feeling the positive emotions associated with it. Allow the imagery to inspire calmness or motivation.

Tips for Developing a Lasting Meditation Practice

Be Patient: Meditation is a skill that grows over time. If your mind wanders, gently bring it back to your point of focus.

Create a Ritual: Choose a specific time each day to meditate, integrating it into your routine.

Experiment: Try different types of meditation to discover what resonates most with you.

Use Tools if Needed: Meditation apps, music, or guided meditations can offer structure and support, especially for beginners.

Embrace Growth: Meditation is not about perfection but about presence. Celebrate each moment of stillness you find.

With so many meditation practices available, it's clear that there is something for everyone, regardless of your preferences or lifestyle. From the simplicity of mindfulness to the depth of Vipassana, and from the movement of yoga to the stillness of Zen, each form provides its own pathway to healing, clarity, and peace. To experience the full range of benefits meditation offers, it's important to explore and experiment with different styles. Whether you're seeking relaxation, personal growth, or spiritual awakening, meditation serves as a transformative tool that can guide you towards a life of presence, compassion, and inner peace.

Start small, be patient, and discover which practice resonates most deeply with you. Through this practice, you cultivate a path to a peaceful and empowered life. With dedication, you will find that meditation is not just a practice but a doorway to living with awareness, compassion, and grace in every moment.

"The ego is like a caterpillar. It must shed its skin to become a butterfly. The caterpillar isn't wrong; it's just not yet fully evolved."[40]

—Ram Dass

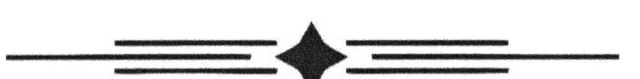

CHAPTER 23

TRANSCENDING THE EGO: THE REBIRTH OF THE TRUE SELF

The ego, often viewed with negativity in many spiritual traditions, plays an essential role in the human experience. It is not inherently *"bad"* or something to be eliminated entirely, but rather something to be understood, transcended, and integrated.

The ego arises as a defense mechanism to help us navigate the world, protect us from external threats, and preserve our sense of identity in a complex, often chaotic environment. Without it, we would struggle to function in the world, to maintain a sense of self, or to differentiate between what is safe and what is harmful. At its core, the ego is our psychological structure that helps us define who we are and where we fit in the world. It develops early in life as a response to survival instincts, shaping itself around experiences, social conditioning, and emotional needs. In this way, it is a product of our life experiences—it holds onto past traumas, defends against perceived threats, and reacts based on learned behaviors.

The ego becomes problematic, however, when it overextends its protective function. Rather than serving as a guide for survival, it becomes rigid, limiting, and often out of touch with the deeper aspects of the self. When we attach too strongly to its defenses, we begin to identify too deeply with our external circumstances, beliefs, and roles. We start to equate who we are with what we have—our job, our possessions, our achievements, or even our social status. This is where it can cause harm because it convinces us that our worth is contingent upon external factors, and it fosters a sense of separation from others and from our deeper, truer selves.

The ego's need for control, validation, and separation leads to suffering. It fuels fear, insecurity, and anxiety because it feels constantly threatened by change, rejection, or failure. As it reinforces these fears, it keeps us trapped in a loop of striving for external approval or material success, believing that these will somehow fill the internal void. To serve our growth, we must transcend its limitations—not by rejecting or annihilating it, but by allowing it to fulfill its protective function and then moving beyond it. Transcending the ego involves recognizing its role, understanding when it is trying to protect us, and learning to trust a deeper, more authentic part of ourselves that is not dependent on external validation or survival instincts.

This shift happens when we stop identifying with the ego and instead view it as a tool that can be used to navigate the world without fully defining who we are.

The Necessity of Ego in Protection

The ego serves as a crucial tool for our survival. It creates boundaries and helps us navigate the complexities of human relationships and societal expectations. It helps us discern what is *"safe"* versus what is *"unsafe,"* and in doing so, it prevents us from harm in a world full of potential dangers. This is why it is often formed in childhood when we are most vulnerable, as a means of protecting ourselves from emotional, physical, and psychological harm. Without this protective layer, we would have no sense of personal safety, no sense of identity, and no mechanism to help us interpret the world around us.

In this sense, it is not an enemy but a necessary aspect of the human experience. It helps us understand who we are in relation to the world and is responsible for keeping us grounded in the practicalities of life. It helps us function as individuals, make decisions, and interact with others in meaningful ways.

The problem arises when the ego becomes overly protective or defensive. It begins to create a false sense of security by holding onto outdated beliefs, emotional wounds, or attachments. It starts to tell us that we are only the roles we play (e.g., *I am a mother, I am a doctor, I am successful*), leading to a narrow, often distorted sense of self. It builds walls around us to protect us from perceived threats, but these walls also isolate us from our true essence and from others.

Transcending the ego does not mean eliminating it; it means going beyond it. It means recognizing that while it serves a vital role in keeping us safe, it does not define who we are at our deepest core. To transcend the ego is to shift from being driven by the ego to observing the ego. When we can step back and watch it's work without identifying with it, we can move beyond its limited perspective and embrace a higher level of consciousness.

This transcendent process involves a deepening of self-awareness and a willingness to let go of the old patterns and defenses that no longer serve us. It means recognizing when the ego is trying to protect us out of fear and choosing to trust in a deeper wisdom. It requires us to be willing to face our deepest fears, insecurities, and vulnerabilities—those parts of ourselves that the ego has tried to shield us from.

As we transcend it, we become more connected to our true self. We begin to operate from a place of love, compassion, and authenticity, rather than from fear, control, and protection. We no longer define ourselves by external circumstances, nor do we feel the need to protect ourselves at all costs. Instead, we trust that our inherent worth is not contingent on external validation or success.

Ego Transcendence—The Birth of the True Self

"The less you identify with the ego, the more free you become. To transcend the ego is to return to your natural state of being."[41] – Osho

The process of transcending the ego is ultimately one of spiritual evolution. As the ego collapses, it makes room for the emergence of the true self—the essence that has always been within us but was obscured by layers of fear, conditioning, and false beliefs.

This true self is not concerned with survival or external validation, but with expressing itself authentically and living in alignment with its higher purpose. This is the *"rebirth"* process that spiritual traditions often speak of—the shedding of the false self and the birth of the true self. This process is not about getting rid of the ego, but about transcending its limited, fear-based influence and integrating it into a larger sense of wholeness and spiritual awareness.

As we move beyond ego-based thinking, we begin to experience life from a higher perspective. We start to recognize that we are not separate from others or from the universe but interconnected with all life. This shift in perception is what allows us to experience true freedom and fulfillment, as we no longer live in constant defense mode, trying to protect a fragile sense of self. Instead, we live from a place of wholeness, trusting that the true self, free of fear and insecurity, is always enough.

In this sense, the ego's collapse is not a loss but a necessary evolution—a vital step in the process of spiritual awakening. It is the death of the false self, making way for the emergence of the true self, and ultimately leading us to a life of greater peace, purpose, and connection. The ego, once transcended, becomes an ally rather than an obstacle—allowing us to engage with the world in a deeper, more authentic way.

Practice: From Ego to Essence

The journey from ego to essence is about shifting from a life ruled by external roles, fears, and defenses to a state of authentic being aligned with your true nature. This path invites you to understand the ego's purpose, recognize its limitations, and transcend it by reconnecting with your essence—your infinite, divine self.

These practices will help you observe it with compassion, dismantle its illusions, and embrace the clarity and freedom of your essence.

Awareness of the Ego's Voice

Develop mindfulness and discern the ego's patterns in your thoughts and actions.

Daily Reflection: At the end of each day, journal moments when you felt defensive, fearful, or overly attached to outcomes. Note the ego's motivations, such as seeking validation, avoiding criticism, or controlling situations.

Naming the ego: Give your ego a playful or symbolic name to separate it from your true self. For example, you might call it *The Protector* or *The Achiever.* When you notice ego-driven thoughts, address it by name with compassion: *Thank you, Protector, but I choose differently.*

Anchoring in the Present Moment

Quiet the ego's chatter by focusing on the present, where the true self resides.

Breath Awareness: Spend a few minutes each morning focusing on your breath. As thoughts arise, gently return to your breathing, observing the ego's attempts to distract you without judgment.

Engaging the Senses: Choose an everyday activity, such as drinking tea or walking, and fully immerse in it. Feel the textures, notice the sounds, and experience each moment without attaching labels or judgments.

Ego-Softening through Gratitude

Shift focus from the ego's fears and lacks to a mindset of abundance and appreciation.

Gratitude Journaling: Write three things each day you're grateful for, focusing on inner qualities or simple joys (e.g., *I'm grateful for my resilience* or *I appreciated the warmth of the sun today*).

Acknowledging Others: Share gratitude directly with someone in your life, reinforcing connection and softening the ego's tendency toward separation.

Shadow Work: Befriending the Ego's Fears

Bring compassion to hidden fears and patterns the ego tries to suppress.

Inner Dialogue: When you feel triggered, close your eyes and ask: *What is the fear or belief beneath this reaction?* Allow the ego's voice to surface and journal the answers.

Compassionate Reassurance: Respond to these fears as you would to a child, offering reassurance and affirming that you are safe and loved beyond external circumstances.

Essence Meditation

Connect directly with your essence, bypassing the ego's distractions.

Visualization: Sit in stillness and imagine a bright light at the center of your chest. With each inhale, visualize this light expanding, representing your true self. With each exhale, imagine shedding a layer of ego-driven fear or identity.

Mantra Practice: Repeat a phrase that aligns with your essence, such as: *I am whole,* or *I am infinite love.* Let it guide your focus back to your essence when distractions arise.

Detaching from Roles and Labels

Release identification with societal or self-imposed roles.

Who Am I? Exercise: Write *Who am I?* at the top of a page. List everything you identify as (e.g., *I am a parent, I am successful).* Then ask: *Who am I without these roles?* Reflect on the qualities that remain.

Role-Free Day: Dedicate a day to stepping outside usual roles. Avoid over-identifying with your job or social status, and spend time exploring your essence through creativity, nature, or stillness.

Embodying Authenticity

Live from your essence by aligning actions and choices with your true self.

Heart Check-In: Before making decisions, ask yourself: *Am I acting from fear (ego) or love (essence)?* Choose actions that reflect your values and authentic desires.

Speak Your Truth: Practice voicing your needs and boundaries honestly without fear of judgment, trusting that your essence thrives in authenticity.

The Mirror of Relationships

Use interactions with others as opportunities for self-discovery and ego transcendence.

Observing Triggers: When someone triggers frustration, jealousy, or fear, ask: *What is this reflecting about my ego's needs or wounds?* Use this awareness to grow instead of reacting.

Conscious Connection: In conversations, practice deep listening. Shift your focus from defending your ego's perspective to truly understanding the other person's essence.

Acts of Surrender

Loosen the ego's need for control and deepen trust in life's flow.

Daily Surrender Practice: Begin each day by affirming: *I release control and trust that life unfolds for my highest good.*

Non-Attachment Exercise: Choose an area of life (e.g., work, relationships) where you feel the need for control. Consciously practice letting go of specific outcomes and observe the results

Aligning with Universal Oneness

Awareness beyond the ego's sense of separation.

Nature Connection: Spend time in nature, observing its interconnectedness. Reflect on how you are a part of this unity, not separate from it.

Compassionate Service: Engage in acts of kindness without expectation of reward, reinforcing the essence of connection and love.

The journey from ego to essence is a profound act of self-discovery, healing, and transformation. These practices help you observe, soften, and transcend the ego's grip, allowing your essence to shine through. In this state, you are free to experience the boundless potential of your existence, living from a place of wholeness rather than limitation.

"Who looks outside, dreams; who looks inside, awakes."[42]

—*Carl Jung*

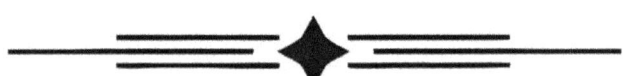

CHAPTER 24

THE EVOLUTION OF SPIRITUALITY: BREAKING DOWN OLD PARADIGMS TO BUILD NEW FOUNDATIONS

The world of spirituality, like any other domain of human consciousness, is in a state of evolution. What once served as guiding lights for countless individuals—manifestation techniques, self-help methods, and even ideas of abundance—are now being questioned. The methods that once promised success and transformation are showing cracks, exposing the truth that they were built on unstable foundations. In our modern era, many are discovering that the approaches that seemed to work in the past were just temporary fixes, not solutions rooted in lasting authenticity.

The old spiritual paradigms were often based on external manifestations and the pursuit of desires—be it wealth, success, or validation. Methods like vision boards, affirmations, and positive thinking are perceived as the keys to happiness and fulfillment. However, these techniques, though helpful in some ways, often ignored deeper emotional traumas and the personal belief systems that had shaped individuals' lives.

The spiritual path, for many, became a constant striving—an endless pursuit of something *"outside"* of themselves to fix a perceived lack. This paradigm focused on external achievements as a measure of spiritual success. People sought to manifest their desires, believing that material abundance or social recognition would solve their deeper issues. In reality, these manifestations merely moved the chairs around in a house built on a shaky, cracked foundation. While external circumstances might shift momentarily, the unresolved trauma, limiting beliefs, and false identities lurking within remained.

The Process of Breaking Down the False Self

Just as a house built on a faulty foundation will eventually collapse, so too will the false self—the identity constructed from wounds, fears, and societal conditioning. The more we cling to outdated spiritual practices that promise quick fixes, the further we move from true healing. What is truly required is a dismantling of the false identity and a return to our authentic essence.

This process of inner work often feels like a traumatic experience. We may feel as though everything is falling apart—relationships, finances, careers, or even our sense of self. But just as in the process of birth, this destruction is necessary to create space for something new. It's like tearing down the walls of a house and pouring a new foundation, not to replace who we are but to reconnect to the essence of what we've always been.

The notion of manifestation often leads to disappointment because it is rooted in the ego's desire for control. When individuals rely on techniques like vision boards or positive affirmations without addressing the underlying emotional blocks and limiting beliefs, they find that the manifestation of external things does not equate to happiness or fulfillment.

This is because external circumstances cannot heal the internal wounds. Manifesting material wealth or success, for example, does not guarantee emotional healing or spiritual growth. A person may manifest financial abundance but still struggle with feelings of inadequacy, loneliness, or fear of losing what they've gained.

The old paradigm of manifestation did not recognize that the root of our desires often lies in trauma, insecurity, or fear. Until we heal these deeper wounds, any success or abundance we manifest will simply be a temporary fix, like putting a new coat of paint on a crumbling house. The path to spiritual growth recognizes that transformation comes from within. True healing requires addressing the foundational trauma and false beliefs that shape our lives. It is about breaking down the old identity and allowing the true self to emerge. This process is messy, uncomfortable, and often painful, but it is necessary for the birth of a more authentic and empowered self.

Instead of focusing on what we want to manifest in the world, we must shift our focus to who we are becoming. The key to this evolution lies in the willingness to sit with discomfort and face the parts of ourselves we've ignored or hidden. When we confront our fears, insecurities, and traumas, we make space for our true essence to emerge—a self that is not defined by external circumstances but by an inner knowing of our worth and purpose.

The New Foundation: Building on Authenticity

As the old paradigms crumble, we are left with the opportunity to rebuild on a more solid foundation—one based on authenticity, self-acceptance, and spiritual alignment. This new foundation is not about seeking external validation or material gain but about aligning with our true essence and allowing it to guide us.

The practice of listening to our souls, as opposed to our fears, is at the heart of this new approach. When we follow our soul's calling, we move away from the ego's need for control and begin to trust the unfolding of life.

This trust is a radical shift from the old way of thinking, where we believed that we needed to force outcomes and control every aspect of our lives. Instead of relying on manifestation techniques that promise external rewards, we begin to embrace the process of inner transformation. This is the real work— purging the lies we've believed about ourselves and allowing the light of truth to emerge. This process may feel like everything is falling apart, but it is in the destruction of the false self that the true self is reborn.

The *"dark nights of the soul"*, once feared and avoided, are now seen for what they truly are—opportunities for deep healing and transformation. The ego's transcendence is not a loss; it is the necessary death of the false self, making room for the emergence of the true self. This rebirth process is not only personal but collective. The world is also going through its own dark night, as the old systems, structures, and paradigms crumble. But just as in individual healing, this collapse is making space for a new way of being, both for individuals and for society as a whole.

The shift in spiritual understanding is underway. The old ways of seeking happiness, fulfillment, and success—through manifestation, external validation, and positive thinking—are giving way to a more profound understanding of inner healing. As we rebuild from the ground up, we are learning that true peace and fulfillment come not from external achievements but from internal transformation. The foundation of our spiritual growth must be laid with authenticity, self-love, and acceptance of all that we are, including the darkness that exists within. When we embrace the full spectrum of our being, we unlock the true power and potential of who we are meant to be.

By letting go of old patterns and beliefs, we make room for the miraculous emergence of our authentic selves—a self that is already whole, already healed, and aligned with the greater truth of the universe. Connecting with our higher self means aligning with the deepest, truest part of our being—beyond ego, fear, or external validation. It is the key to genuine transformation, guiding us toward authenticity, inner peace, and a life in alignment with our soul's purpose.

This connection opens the door to profound wisdom, empowering us to live with clarity, compassion, and a deep sense of fulfillment. This is the new spiritual paradigm: one rooted in love, authenticity, and the deep knowing that we are enough as we are.

A Shift from Practices to Presence

In the evolution of spirituality, we are moving away from the rigid adherence to specific practices and techniques and embracing a deeper, more organic approach that aligns with our true essence. The old spiritual paradigms often emphasized the importance of daily practices, visualization exercises, or manifestation techniques to *"achieve"* personal growth or external success. These practices, while helpful in some contexts, were often rooted in the belief that we must *"do"* something in order to attain spiritual enlightenment or inner peace.

However, as we shift toward a more authentic and holistic understanding of spirituality, we begin to realize that spiritual growth is not something to be *"achieved"* but something to be recognized and allowed. The true essence of spirituality lies in the presence of our being, rather than the actions we take.

The old notion of forcing or manipulating our reality through specific practices is being replaced by an understanding that spiritual transformation arises from within—through self-awareness, surrender, and a willingness to embrace who we truly are.

The Illusion of Practices

Practices, such as visualization, affirmations, or rituals, were often viewed as essential tools for manifesting desired outcomes—be it success, healing, or personal transformation. While these practices can be useful in certain stages of spiritual growth, they often become a distraction if the underlying beliefs and wounds remain unaddressed.

In the past, many people relied on practices as a means of fixing their lives or achieving a sense of completeness. Yet, these practices frequently missed the deeper work of releasing the false self and reconnecting with our true essence. The reality is that no amount of affirmation, visualization, or ritual can replace the necessary work of transforming the inner landscape—the emotional wounds, limiting beliefs, and conditioned identities that shape our lives.

When we focus only on practices, we risk reinforcing the idea that something is missing within us, and that we need to *"do"* something to be complete. The truth, however, is that we are already whole. The only thing that needs to change is our relationship to our own being.

Shifting from "Doing" to "Being"

The new spiritual paradigm encourages a shift from doing to being. This doesn't mean abandoning all practices but recognizing that true spiritual growth emerges from an inner alignment rather than external effort. The focus is no longer on what we need to do to change our circumstances or manifest external results, but on who we are becoming.

The process of spiritual transformation is no longer about forcing outcomes through practices or following specific rules. It's about allowing the unfolding of our true selves.

When we align with our authentic essence, we no longer need to strive to *"make"* things happen. We begin to live in harmony with life, trusting that the natural flow of existence will guide us. The key is surrender—letting go of control, releasing the need for external validation, and trusting that everything we need is already within us.

This shift represents a radical change in how we approach spirituality. The old methods taught us that we had to *"manifest"* or *"create"* our spiritual path through external actions. In contrast, the new understanding invites us to trust the process, to be present with ourselves, and to embrace the truth that our inherent worth and purpose do not need to be achieved—they are already part of who we are. Rather than focusing on the perfection of practices, the new spiritual system encourages us to cultivate presence. Presence is the practice of being fully engaged in the present moment, without judgment, without striving, and without the need to fix anything. It is through presence that we become aware of the underlying truths that guide us toward authentic transformation.

Instead of focusing on practices to control or manifest specific outcomes, you are invited to trust the inner journey of self-discovery. The collapse of the old egoic self, the breaking down of false identities, and the healing of deep-seated traumas are all part of this transformative process.

There is no need to force change through rituals or techniques; the true spiritual evolution happens organically when we stop resisting what is and allow ourselves to be guided by our soul's wisdom. Practices are no longer viewed as the means to an end. Instead, we understand that true spiritual growth arises from within when we stop trying to control our outcomes and start embracing the process of self-discovery. This approach to spirituality does not negate the importance of mindful practices but places them in their rightful context: not as tools to fix what is broken but as expressions of our already whole being.

The real transformation lies in our willingness to trust in the process, embrace our imperfections, and be present with the moment. By shifting from a mindset of *"doing"* to one of *"being,"* we reconnect with our true essence and allow the natural unfolding of our spiritual evolution. Presence allows us to sit with discomfort, to face our fears, and to allow the layers of our false identity to dissolve naturally. When we are present with our emotions, our thoughts, and our experiences, we no longer see them as obstacles to be overcome but as aspects of our journey that hold wisdom.

This presence, this full acceptance of ourselves as we are, becomes the true practice of the new spiritual paradigm.

NOTES

1. Chödrön, Pema. *When Things Fall Apart: Heart Advice for Difficult Times.* Shambhala, 2000.

2. Krishnamurti, Jiddu. *The First and Last Freedom.* Harper & Row, 1954.

3. Yogananda, Paramahansa. *The Essence of Self-Realization.* Self-Realization Fellowship, 1989.

4. Teilhard de Chardin, Pierre. *The Phenomenon of Man.* Harper & Row, 1959.

5. Charles Darwin, *On the Origin of Species* (London: John Murray, 1859).

6. Deepak Chopra, *The Book of Secrets: Unlocking the Hidden Dimensions of Your Life* (New York: Three Rivers Press, 2004), 88.

7. Buddha, *The Dhammapada*, trans. Eknath Easwaran (Tomales, CA: Nilgiri Press, 2007), 45.

8. Sadhguru, *Inner Engineering: A Yogi's Guide to Joy* (New York: Penguin Random House, 2016), 45.

9. Rumi, *The Essential Rumi*, trans. Coleman Barks (New York: HarperSanFrancisco, 1995), 129.

10. Lao Tzu, *Tao Te Ching*, trans. Stephen Mitchell (New York: HarperCollins, 1988), 78.

11. Mahatma Gandhi, *The Collected Works of Mahatma Gandhi*, vol. 10 (Ahmedabad: Navajivan Publishing House, 1958), 250.

12. Eckhart Tolle, *A New Earth: Awakening to Your Life's Purpose* (New York: Penguin Group, 2005), 123.

13. Martin Luther King Jr., *Strength to Love* (Philadelphia: Harper & Row, 1963), 46.

14. Dalai Lama, *The Art of Happiness* (New York: Riverhead Books, 1998), 98.

15. Einstein, *The World As I See It* (New York: Philosophical Library, 1949).

16. Cannon, *The Convoluted Universe: Book One* (Fairfield, IA: Ozark Mountain Publishing, 2001).

17. Williamson, Marianne. *A Return to Love: Reflections on the Principles of "A Course in Miracles"*. New York: HarperCollins, 1992.

18. Blavatsky, Helena. *The Secret Doctrine*. Vol. 1. Theosophical Publishing House, 1888.

19. Rumi. *The Essential Rumi*, translated by Coleman Barks. HarperOne, 1995.

20. Laozi, *Tao Te Ching*, trans. Stephen Mitchell (New York: HarperCollins, 1988), 74.

21. Rumi, *The Essential Rumi*, trans. Coleman Barks (New York: HarperCollins, 1995), 32.

22. Kabat-Zinn, Jon. *Wherever You Go, There You Are: Mindfulness Meditation in Everyday Life*. New York: Hyperion, 1994.

23. Eckhart Tolle, *The Power of Now: A Guide to Spiritual Enlightenment* (Novato, CA: New World Library, 1999), 65.

24. Mahatma Gandhi, *The Collected Works of Mahatma Gandhi*, vol. 5 (Ahmedabad: Navajivan Publishing House, 1958), 245.

25. Dyer, Wayne. *The Power of Intention: Learning to Co-create Your World Your Way*. Carlsbad, CA: Hay House, 2004.

26. Brown, Brené. *Rising Strong: The Reckoning. The Rumble. The Revolution*. Spiegel & Grau, 2015.

27. Nin, Anaïs. *Seduction of the Minotaur*. Harcourt Brace Jovanovich, 1961

28. Jung, Carl. *Psychological Aspects of the Persona*. 1953.

29. Hay, Louise. *You Can Heal Your Life*. Hay House, 1984.

30. Epictetus. *The Enchiridion*. Translated by Elizabeth Carter. 1758. Reprint, Dover Publications, 2004.

31. Gaur, Bhavya. *The Akashic Records: Unlock the Infinite Power, Wisdom, and Energy of the Universe*.

32. Edgar Cayce, *The Edgar Cayce Reader* (New York: Macmillan, 1965), 152.

33. Helena Petrovna Blavatsky, *The Secret Doctrine* (Adyar, India: The Theosophical Publishing House, 1888), 101.

34. Alfred Percy Sinnett, *The Occult World* (London: Trübner & Co., 1888), 87.

35. Rudolf Steiner, *The Fifth Gospel* (Hudson, NY: Anthroposophic Press, 1999), 23.

36. Usui, Mikao. *Reiki: The Healing Touch*. Translated by Bronwen and Frans Stiene. Waiora International, 1999.

37. Hanh, Thich Nhat. *The Heart of the Buddha's Teaching: Transforming Suffering into Peace, Joy, and Liberation*. Broadway Books, 1998.

38. Vivekananda, Swami. *The Complete Works of Swami Vivekananda*. Vol. 1. Advaita Ashrama, 1997.

39. Ram Dass. *Be Here Now*. Lama Foundation, 1971.

40. Ram Dass. *Polishing the Mirror: How to Live from Your Spiritual Heart*. HarperOne, 2013.

41. Osho. *The Book of Secrets: 112 Meditations to Discover the Mystery Within*. St. Martin's Griffin, 2001.

42. Jung, Carl. *Psychological Reflections: An Anthology of His Writings*. Edited by Jolande Jacobi. Princeton University Press, 1978.

ABOUT THE AUTHOR

Ioana Aura Munteanu holds a degree in Civil Law and has pursued additional studies in Indigenous Relations at the University of Alberta. With over 25 years of experience across diverse traditions, she brings together ancient wisdom and modern science to guide others on the path of personal transformation. Born in Romania, she now lives in Alberta, Canada, with her husband and their three children.

www.ingramcontent.com/pod-product-compliance
Lightning Source LLC
Chambersburg PA
CBHW051133120626
46547CB00012B/783